INTERMITTENT FASTING FOR WOMEN OVER 50

THE 3-STEP TRANSFORMATIONAL FORMULA TO
MELT FAT IN LESS THAN 27 DAYS

NAOMI LINDSEY

© Copyright 2023 Naomi Lindsey - All rights reserved.

The content contained within this book may not be reproduced, duplicated or transmitted without direct written permission from the author or the publisher.

Under no circumstances will any blame or legal responsibility be held against the publisher, or author, for any damages, reparation, or monetary loss due to the information contained within this book. Either directly or indirectly. You are responsible for your own choices, actions, and results.

Legal Notice:

This book is copyright protected. This book is only for personal use. You cannot amend, distribute, sell, use, quote or paraphrase any part, or the content within this book, without the consent of the author or publisher.

Disclaimer Notice:

Please note the information contained within this document is for educational and entertainment purposes only. All effort has been executed to present accurate, up-to-date, and reliable, complete information. No warranties of any kind are declared or implied. Readers acknowledge that the author is not engaging in the rendering of legal, financial, medical or professional advice. The content within this book has been derived from various sources. Please consult a licensed professional before attempting any techniques outlined in this book.

By reading this document, the reader agrees that under no circumstances is the author responsible for any losses, direct or indirect, which are incurred as a result of the use of the information contained within this document, including, but not limited to, — errors, omissions, or inaccuracies.

This book is dedicated to my mother Elizabeth-Anne Mary Ryner, who taught me how to fast, what to eat, and when to eat and brought me up in Love on the True Vine.

CONTENTS

Introduction	ix
1. INTERMITTENT FASTING: YOUR BRIDGE TO YOUR IDEAL BODY	1
From Fat to Fit	2
So, What Exactly is Intermittent Fasting?	2
How: The Consequential Autophagy and Physical Changes	3
Undo Those Destructive Beliefs	4
Compelling Benefits of Intermittent Fasting	7
Women are Winning and Regaining Control of Their Lives	11
2. HORMONE HARMONIZATION & RESURRECTING THE 12 SYSTEMS	16
The ME-NO-Pause Story	16
Menopausal Transitions and Expected Developments	17
Habitudes to Harmonize Your Hormones Like Honey	21
Intermittent Fasting Harmonizes These Hormones	37
Intermittent Fasting Resurrects the 12 Systems	38
Pre- And Post-Menopausal Women with Breast Cancers	42
Harmonize Hormones Naturally	43
3. BREAKING THROUGH THE BARRIERS	46
Reimaging	47
Reality Check - Current Routine Evaluation	47
Sleep Hygiene	48
Stress Mitigation	51
Synergistic Relationships	54
Eating Quality	55
Exercise Regime	56
Spiritual Fulfillment	57
Visual Inspiration	58
Conquer Overeating	60

4. **CONSCIOUS INTERMITTENT FASTING FORMULA: WHEN** — 64
   - Fasting Methods — 65
   - Intermittent Fasting During Peri-menopause — 71
   - Intermittent Fasting During All Phases — 72
   - Hydration Formula — 73
   - The Jet Lag Relief — 74
   - Celebratory Events — 74
   - Medication And Supplements While Fasting — 75
   - Common Fasting Mistakes — 76

5. **CONSCIOUS FEASTING: WHAT TO EAT** — 78
   - Breaking a Short Fast — 79
   - Breaking an Extended Fast — 79
   - Foods To Avoid After a Fast — 80
   - Eradicate Bloating — 80
   - Regeneration Formula After Cancer — 81
   - Evaluate Your Food Supply — 83
   - Mediterranean Style — 85
   - Planned Foods to Have Available Ahead of Intermittent Fasting — 86
   - Substitutes, Sugar and Sweeteners — 87

6. **DANCE TO THE RIGHT TUNE: ENOUGH IS ENOUGH** — 90
   - Increasing Calcium Absorption: What, How and When — 91
   - Recommendations for Increasing Calcium Absorption — 101
   - Exercise is Fictitious — 103
   - 7-day Challenge — 104

7. **FEASTING FORMULA** — 113
   - Eating Order — 113
   - Meal Schedule — 115
   - Food Combination Formula — 116
   - Food Combinations To Acknowledge — 120

8. **CONSCIOUS CELEBRATION** — 122
   - Intuitive Awareness — 122
   - Increased Financial Gain — 123
   - Physical Rewards — 123
   - Psychological Stimulation — 124

Tracking	124
Celebrate Wins Exuberantly	125
More Empowerment To You	128
9. BONUS: MEDITERRANEAN RECIPES	131
Added Bonus: Finger-lickin' Indian Recipes	161
Accountability	171
Notes	173
About Naomi Lindsey	181

INTRODUCTION

Let's give ourselves a minute and think of something hard to lose. Money? Ah, no. Hair? Definitely, no. Relationships? Okay, it is getting awkward.

Weight? Absolutely!

Why is weight so hard to lose? So hard that you often end up accepting it as a part of your life. You made peace with the fact that you can probably never fit yourself into that cute little black dress or can never flaunt a crop top and that XXL is the new 'S.' You are even okay with not looking at yourself in a mirror. I had been there and done all that and even more.

You successfully somehow managed to get through your 'younger' days. But things start getting worse when you touch your 50s when peri-menopause, menopause, and post-menopause symptoms start hitting you like a multi-vehicle pile-up on a highway. You become prone to irritable bowel syndrome (IBS), colitis, inflammatory bowel disease (IBD), obesity, diabetes, high cholesterol, headache, anxiety issues, mood swings, and everything else you have probably only heard of on a health channel. Why? Because of the stubborn pounds that, like an uninvited guest, won't go away. Add your non-stop cycle of eating and drinking day and night.

I remember how I ended up eating and drinking more because I felt terrible about my body weight. And then that unconscious consumption added pounds to my body, blessing me with chronic illnesses. A vicious cycle of which I was once a part.

I'll be frank. I am not even the right person to talk to about losing weight. Exercising was never my thing. Getting fatter was one of my talents from birth. Even my desk job and sedentary lifestyle contributed to it. I exhausted all my waking hours at work, meeting deadlines. I was in a toxic relationship with weight, none of us was enjoying the company of each other, yet divorce was out of the question. This relationship with ever-growing fat soon manifested in mood swings, headaches, migraines, dark circles, arthritis, and cardiovascular diseases, and I'll stop it here.

You see, weight loss was challenging for me. But I did achieve it. And that gives me every reason to talk with you. Of course, there always will be enough reasons not to achieve a particular thing. But there will also be one reason good enough that will make you push your boundaries, challenge your limits, and go all in. That one reason for me was my budget. It was not a challenging calculation to realize that I had spent too much on medication only to get dull and puffy eyes, drooping cheeks, deep-set wrinkles, an unhealthy fatty body, a round belly, cellulite, brittle nails, and scaly skin.

Don't get me wrong. A round belly and fat body are beautiful, extremely beautiful. What is not beautiful is the disease-causing stubborn fat that won't budge no matter what. That's when I knew I would draw the line.

And, you know what? Not only do I flaunt a healthy body now, but my finances have also significantly improved. I no longer binge and spend extravagantly on food. I don't have to load my body with all those expensive medicinal chemicals.

I want to share what I learned late with women in their 50s. I still remember how I dreaded going to beaches because of my restricted mobility. It took a while to admit I had trouble walking, even for a few meters in a stretch. Finally, my husband and I decided to go for a walk one fine evening. You know the weather is delightful, the sky is pink, the breeze is pleasant, and you give in to your temptations? He suggested that we go outside to get some fresh air. Of course, I said yes without giving it a second thought. But, girl, was that a wrong call? It took all my willpower, lung power, and horsepower to pull that massive chunk of fat uphill. And I felt ashamed to reveal to him that I was struggling because that ripped hunk was clearly on a stroll while I was desperately wheezing for the defibrillator, yet I was clearly in the stage of denial then. Frustrated, I even postponed the plans to celebrate our wedding anniversary on the beach. But frustration was soon followed by acceptance and acceptance by action, and here I am now.

My body is better balanced and toned; I have never looked this young and healthy. How? I only followed a simple process called intermittent fasting. Fasting is not new. Therapeutically used since the 5th century BC, the Greek physician Hippocrates II recommended abstinence from drinks and food to patients suffering from illness. But the idea of fasting was alien to me. What? Not eat? Me? Never? How did I ever give in to such a concept? But that's what I did. And let me break it down for you. It is not rocket science, just a bit of biology applied here and there.

During our time together, I will first introduce you to intermittent fasting. As you might have heard, it is way different, systematic, and result-oriented than regular dieting. I will then discuss how intermittent fasting helps you balance your hormones. Finally, once we have understood the basics, I will help you break the barriers and prepare you for your transformational journey.

I will share a fasting formula with you. Then, I'll discuss what, when, and how to eat. I'll also help you incorporate strength training with intermittent fasting. And

I will also talk about my journey and how I kept working on it even when there was no light at the tunnel's beginning. But I soon found my way out to paradise, and you can too.

So, without further ado, let's jump in with both feet and discover how intermittent fasting can help you melt fat. I am a living case study who successfully lost 100 lbs; it took time. But I can help you lose pounds in twenty-seven transformational days.

Let's delve deeper. Shall we?

1

INTERMITTENT FASTING: YOUR BRIDGE TO YOUR IDEAL BODY

Your body is a temple. While the temptation to go with the flow and live each day to the fullest may seem enticing, often, that is not the most conducive way to live life. Those looking to make positive changes in their lifestyle are often too quick to jump into gym activities, cycling, running, or even swimming. While all these activities are legitimate and helpful, taking up commitments like intermittent fasting gets pushed to one side.

I have often been met with confused and skeptical faces when I advocate practices like intermittent fasting. The dominant image is that of an unhealthy hacky method that requires one to give up food. Losing interest soon follows this initial apprehension, which is a real shame because intermittent fasting, a.k.a. IF, simply works!

I choose to educate on the benefits of timed meals to dispel the lousy reputation of intermittent fasting. If you've reached a point where it's a little too late to make a change, I guarantee you, you haven't! On the other hand, nobody is ever too far gone if they're willing to take up the challenge and work smartly towards improvement. We only get one body, so why not do our best to care for it? Let me illustrate how easy it is to do and achieve quick and lasting results with this practice.

From Fat to Fit

You name it; I had it. What, you ask? Almost every lifestyle disease conceivable to man. At age 50, my years of not caring for my body took a genuine and alarming toll on me and greatly affected my everyday life. The necessities of my job and several other factors had me chair bound, unable to get any legitimate exercise into my daily routine. As a result, I was gaining weight so rapidly that I didn't know possible.

Things weren't the same as they used to be when I was younger. After each diet, I'd get on the scale and see that I had made no significant change except for a weight increase. Exercising drained and sapped me rather than gave me the energy promised.

As I grew older, hormonal imbalances contributed significantly to my rapid weight gain. So, it was no surprise when the doctor declared that I was obese and had several health conditions that required prompt attention. My couch potato lifestyle had caught up to me in my later years, and I was paying a heavy toll. Looking in the mirror at myself, I felt nothing but shame and loathing. But enough was enough. I had to get out of this slump. At this point in my life, I found and began to practice intermittent fasting. It did not involve any strenuous exercises.

And believe me. Any movement was strenuous to me at this point. Not only did it help structure my life, but it also soon made me healthier too! Just because I was older than most didn't mean I could give up on myself. I love myself and would like to be here for a long time. So, with a better-late-than-never attitude, I changed my lifestyle. With intermittent fasting, I was able to do just that.

So, What Exactly is Intermittent Fasting?

What you consume, when you ingest it, and how much food you consume are significant. While eating may seem like a practice done for the sake of eating, the quality of nourishment dramatically depends on you regulating your food intake rigorously. While intermittent fasting may sound scary and uncomfortable, it does not have to be. It is any voluntary period during the day when you abstain from food. It is not referred to as a diet because it does not specify what to eat. However, since food is the body's building block, and if you're looking to reap better health benefits, it will do wonders to incorporate authentic, nutritious, natural, and whole colorful foods.

Intermittent fasting is about eating less often, skipping meals, and eliminating snacks. Refrain from keeping your body stuffed with food. The longer the fasting hours are, the better, 16 hours, 18 hours, or 22 hours, whatever works for you. Transitioning too fast could have some adverse effects. Conveniently start by skipping one meal, be it dinner or breakfast. Then if you can do that, go for longer. Intermittent fasting does not mean skipping all your meals. Instead, it means appropriately regulating what you eat and being aware of how your stomach and overall body feel. This strategy allows the body to use the body fat stored as calories and gives it time to rest and digest the food eaten before it breaks the fast.

How: The Consequential Autophagy and Physical Changes

Rather than defining what to eat, intermittent fasting is more interested in the 'when' of everything. However, there is a very legitimate science to back up the efficacy of intermittent fasting. The reason why IF works is because of this body process called autophagy. Autophagy is the body engaging its sustainability system where it recycles, processes, and removes damaged components like impaired DNA, dysfunctional proteins, and other bodily debris.

Awarded the Nobel Prize for his path-breaking findings on how cells recycle themselves through this process of autophagy, Japanese biologist Yoshinori Ohsumi conducted a study in 2016. He showed that it was a legitimate and excellent process that can work alongside other bodily functions that remove entire cells and significantly damaged cells in a process called apoptosis, defined as programmed cell death.

Stimulated by the appropriate trigger, cells that become a threat to survival self-destruct. These are cells infected by viruses and bacteria, cancer cells, and normal cells that helpfully produce antibodies. Radiation, heat, toxins, nutrient removal, and hormones can also trigger normal cells.

Autophagy rapidly increases the number of new and vibrant cells to repopulate the cells removed during apoptosis. These repopulating stem cells regenerate organ tissue and have intense effects on the organ systems of our body. Moreover, this restoration and regeneration are all activated and enhanced in the fasted state.

Autophagy also removes damaged fibroblasts and activates stem cells that help produce stronger fibroblasts. Fibroblasts are a type of fibrous cellular material that supports and contributes to forming connective tissues that connect tissues and organs in the body. In addition, they create new extracellular matrices such as fibrous collagen and elastin, ground substances, and adhesive proteins like fibronectin and laminin. As we know, collagen is terrific for the body and aids strength, force transmission, mobility, and stability. This way, IF makes workouts more effective.

Undo Those Destructive Beliefs

Several myths plague society as we know it and prevent us from taking meaningful steps against issues that can be dealt with adequately. The first myth is that older women should relegate themselves to living with increased and rapid weight gain as it is just a natural part of life and a natural part of growing older.

I very much disagree. I refused to be subpar. I wanted to be optimal! So, with celebrities and iconic figures swearing by this technique, I will now address and subsequently 'bust' all myths most often associated with Intermittent fasting:

By skipping breakfast, you gain more weight

Really? Is eating breakfast the most important meal of the day? It is not. People think that if you skip breakfast, you'll be greedy for the rest of the day. Then you give in to your cravings, eat all day, and gain weight. Science does not support this claim. Studies conducted on as many as 100+ test subjects have shown that amongst overweight and obese adults, there is no real difference between those who eat breakfast and those who do not. Breakfast might benefit some, but only some. So, take this myth with a grain of salt.

Eating more frequently boosts one's metabolism

Some believe that if you eat more, you increase your rate of metabolism, which in turn makes you lose more calories. When you digest your meals, you burn some calories via the thermic effect of food. Studies have shown no significant increase or decrease in calories burnt based on meal frequency. It has more to do with what you eat than when you eat.

Frequent meals make you shrink

Since eating more doesn't boost one's metabolism, the idea that if you eat more frequently, you will lose more weight is very flawed. For example, studies tested people who ate six meals daily and displayed no difference in metabolism and weight loss from those who ate three. Furthermore, there was no difference in fat loss or even appetite. Hence, there is no direct correlation between frequent meals and losing weight.

Your brain requires constant dietary sugar for optimal output

Glucose is not the only fuel your brain can use to function. Your own body can quickly produce the glucose it needs through a process called gluconeogenesis. Ketone bodies produced by your body can also feed parts of your brain, significantly reducing this need or craving for sugar. You are a sugar burner if you get exhausted or shaky from a lack of glucose. Burning sugar means not burning fat in your diet or melting fat. Intermittent fasting hastens your switch to fat burning.

Ramps up overeating

Not true. Intermittent fasting allocates an eating window to regulate previously abusive food habits easily. Therefore, assimilating quality food and portion control improves fasting results.

Intermittent fasting is the saviour for all

While it works for most, you must remember that certain persons cannot do intermittent fasting for medical and other reasons. For example, those with a history of eating disorders, underweight, or those in a weakened and frail body must not engage in IF as it would cause adverse effects. Otherwise, there is no ethnicity or age cap. Intermitting fasting is possible as long as you have an able body and a sound mind.

Impairs your mental senses

Intermittent fasting does not hamper one's mental alertness or focus. However, if you are new to the process and anticipate a temporary drop in your mental alertness and focus, start with a natural 12-hour fast. Preparation will give your body the time to adjust to this change.

Restricting water intake is a normal part of intermittent fasting

Completely false! Rather than decreasing or limiting your water intake, during the fasting period, you must increase your water intake. With Intermittent fasting, drinking water is encouraged because it does wonders to clean your intestines, reduce your appetite, and prevent headaches and constipation.

CATAPULTS your body into starvation

Starvation means suffering or death caused by lack of food, extreme hunger, and famine. In starvation mode, your body's metabolism shuts down, preventing you from burning fat. That is because long-term calorie restriction reduces the number of calories you burn daily and, in turn, reduces your metabolism. However, there is no link between IF and reducing your burnt calories because short-term fasting does not make your body go into starvation mode. It does quite the opposite, where your metabolism increases during fasts for up to 48 hours. Since this is intermittent fasting and not prolonged fasting, there is no starvation mode activation.

Especially in this age of mass media, the false can easily overshadow the real and make you miss out on such a dynamic practice. I have seen the result of intermittent fasting in my life and would advocate it to anyone hoping to make lasting positive changes in their lives.

Compelling Benefits of Intermittent Fasting

This inexhaustive list of myths I have dispelled has clued you in on the various excellent benefits. Here is further insight.

OPTIMIZES your body's operation

There are various changes your body undergoes when you take up intermittent fasting. For one, the blood levels of your insulin drop significantly, facilitating fat burning. Undertaking IF increases your Human Growth Hormone (HGH) levels dramatically. Higher levels of HGH promote muscle gain. Finally, during the fast, your body induces critical cellular repair processes like purging waste from your cells.

DRIVES WEIGHT LOSS and melts visceral fat

Many people who practice intermittent fasting do it for weight loss. They will eat fewer meals than usual, significantly lowering their calorie intake. IF additionally enhances hormone function that facilitates weight loss. Body fat is broken down faster and used for energy. Short-term IF increases your metabolic rate and helps burn more calories. So, intermittent fasting reduces your calories while increasing your metabolic rate. A research experiment in 2014 showed that IF could cause over 3-4% weight loss over a mere 3-24 weeks.

REDUCES and Reverses risk for type-2 diabetes

In recent decades, type-2 diabetes has become very common. In type-2 diabetes, the pancreas cannot produce enough insulin or work satisfactorily, resulting in a lack of insulin, insulin resistance, and high blood sugar. Reducing your sugar intake and, by extension, lowering your blood sugar levels protects you against type-2 diabetes. Studies have tested and proven that during the process of IF, people with a pre-diabetic body show reduced blood sugar levels of about 3-6% over 8-12 weeks. Further research even showed that IF protects against diabetic retinopathy, a complication that sometimes leads to blindness.

REDUCES inflammation and oxidative stress

Oxidative stress contributes to aging. It is an imbalance between antioxidants and free radical activity in the body. For example, the same chemical process causes iron to rust and fruit to rot because the substance loses electrons and gains oxygen. Damage to DNA, lipids, and proteins that comprise a large part of the body leads to many diseases. These include inflammatory conditions, neurogenerative diseases such as Alzheimer's and Parkinson's, hypertension, heart disease, atherosclerosis, diabetes, and cancer. Studies show that IF enhances the body's oxidative stress resistance and dries inflammation.

A MIRACLE RESTORATION for heart health

Intermittent fasting has a significant effect on risk factors associated with heart disease. It improves blood sugar levels, blood pressure, triglycerides, total and LDL (bad) cholesterol, and inflammatory markers. Although scientists did most of the research in animal studies, you must recognize the implications of this research.

ACCELERATES cellular repair processes

While fasting, the autophagy process is booted, and cellular waste removal and recycling occur. The cells initiate autophagy when the environment becomes challenging to the cells because the nutrient source is low. They start by recycling existing misfunctioned organelles and proteins to obtain nutrients. Then, with the help of enzymes and acids, the lysosomes eat old cellular components and unneeded large molecules, including nucleic acid, sugars, and proteins. Lysosomes are organelles that dispose of waste by digesting materials outside the cell. Autophagy is the digestion of the material outside the cell.

These digestive machines destroy invading pathogens such as viruses and bacteria. When cells are in excess, worn out, or beyond repair, these lysosomes assist the cellular garbage in self-destruction, breaking them down into raw materials. The by-products of lysosomal digestion are amino acids and nucleotides. These raw materials are recycled and combined into the functional cell as new cellular components.

During the inventory, malfunctioning proteins are sorted and labeled with a small regulatory protein called ubiquitin, found in eukaryotic cells. Then, unique lipid components near the harmful proteins assemble around the cellular garbage to form vesicles called autophagosomes.

These autophagosomes fuse with lysosomes. The lysosomes use their digestive enzymes to break down and recycle the contents. Autophagosomes can even bundle entire organelles and fuse with lysosomes to degrade insufficient mitochondria. This autophagy process, called mitophagy, destroys old and dysfunctional mitochondria within cells. With age, the body loses its ability to execute this process resulting in neurodegenerative diseases. Efficient mitophagy also eliminates damaged cells from cardiovascular cells. Conversely, faulty mitochondria lead to cell death and, eventually, the death of a person. Therefore, this mitophagy process is critical to sustaining optimal cellular health and attaining healthy aging and longevity.

Autophagy prevents and fights neurodegenerative diseases such as Alzheimer's, Huntington's, and Parkinson's disease and...

Restrains and fights cancer

Cancer cells are the uncontrolled creation of new mitochondria from the division of existing mitochondria. Therefore, they also need to oxygenate themselves to create new mitochondria from the division of existing ones.

As the cell is dividing, it can produce complex proteins and other molecules recognized by the immune system by breaking down small peptides and putting them on the cell surface. Although the immune system can identify these mutations, it is not vigorous enough to create enough cells to create receptors to recognize the tumor. Therefore, the growth of tumors can overcome the small impact the immune response might have on killing any tumor cells. Plus, for a tumor cell to survive and grow, it develops specific properties that can suppress the local immune response to make molecules like Transforming Growth Factor Beta. TGFβ is the discharge of small signal proteins that control the overabundance of physiological and pathological processes during the formation and development of cancer cells. These cells fail to respond to cell cycle signaling, resulting in unregulated growth. As a result, they can leave the site of origin and travel and grow unregulated elsewhere.

So putting selective pressure on these cells through intermittent fasting that inhibits mitochondrial function can lead to their death. Mitophagy ensures the elimination of damaged mitochondria. Fasting has repeatedly shown several beneficial effects on metabolism that reduce cancer risk. Some research evidence also shows that fasting reduces various side effects of chemotherapy in humans.

EXTENDS your lifespan

Let's look at an exhaustive list of what IF does: it melts fat, promotes gut health, creates metabolic flexibility, enhances mitochondrial health, cleans defective cells and other excellent benefits of autophagy, boosts brain health, strengthens immunity, and slows down aging. So, it's no wonder that IF will extend your lifespan. And this long, healthy optimal life is a blessing instead of the curse of dying longer.

OTHER THAN THE BIOLOGICAL REALM, I gained time to think for myself. One thing missing from my world was a spiritual purpose; chasing money threw my life into chaos. So, I started reading my Bible and praying every morning. Following that was my need to declutter my wardrobe, then my garage, and next, I organized my house and my entire household. For once, I set clear boundaries in my relationships and cleared my diary to incorporate relaxation. Now, my family and I take walks, eat dinner together, and express love for each other. These serendipitous rewards blossom into sweet sleep, peace, and rest. Now my conscience is purged; I have no condemnation, regrets, shame, or guilt. I am at peace with myself. The love keeps coming, and this butterfly is still flying high. I am genuinely in love and full of gratitude. Do you believe that I am learning to play the guitar now? It's your turn.

Women are Winning and Regaining Control of Their Lives

Gaining fat is unprecedented regardless of age, ethnicity, or body type. You can never guess when it changes your body so much that your daily life gets disrupted. But, as unlikely as it seems, there is a way around it. The following stories will take you along the journey of 3 different women, at various stages of their lives, on their wellness quest, and introduce you to one common habit that worked for them all!

1. Peri-menopause: Amelda Perkins

Ever since she was a little girl, Amelda was on the chubby side. She was comfortable and happy with her body as long as the scale didn't cross 200 pounds. However, Amelda always felt the need to be fitter. Diet routines would emerge and fade away from her life like floating clouds. At 26, she was a mother of three. Her life changed direction, and she gracefully accepted the weight gain that came with it. Once she turned 30, the little girl inside her wanted to feel fit again, so she started running. Soon enough, she participated in marathons which led to a positive change; she lost weight and felt more confident.

But life was unpredictable - Amelda developed a stress fracture on her right foot and had to put on a cast for three months. Then, all the body fat found its way back to her. During this time, she weighed 189 pounds; Amelda couldn't help but feel despair wash over her.

Things changed when, in 2019, she had a chance conversation with her gynecologist about intermittent fasting. Amelda was apprehensive about trying this out. It seemed like a scheme that offered unrealistic results. However, after conducting her research, convincing evidence persuaded her that intermittent fasting was a scientifically proven method for weight loss.

Amelda started slowly but was consistent. Simple changes like having dinner by 19:00hrs and breakfast at 10:00hrs the next day without snacking in between started working for her. Soon she decided to skip lunch, a significant change, but her body adapted well. The next step she took on was exercising along with intermittent fasting!

"I used the same tenacity and perseverance to start and grow my business. It took time to start earning an income that exceeded my monthly bills. However, my creative mindset kept me inspired and engaged. I finally quit my day job and am excelling in business. Who knew this lifestyle change would have such a stimulating, dynamic effect? Intermittent fasting freed up my time, and I still enjoy an exciting work life balance."

For years, Amelda has gotten better in health and well-being. Intermittent fasting is her way of life now, and she labels it as her best-kept secret for a healthy life!

2. Menopause: Kamal Goyal

At 50, Kamal was diagnosed with pre-diabetes and Non-Alcoholic Fatty Liver. Unfortunately, Kamal's life history had an imprint of struggles with weight loss. Different diets, exercise regimes, and gym subscriptions were part and parcel of Kamal's life. Yet, none of these ever showed any lasting results.

So, at 50, with deteriorating health and a history of weight issues, Kamal stumbled upon the intermittent fasting method. She was intrigued by this idea and incorporated it soon enough. She started with a 16:8 method and then increased her fasting to 19 hours. The positive changes in her body amazed her. Besides weight loss, Kamal's blood sugar and liver enzymes were more regulated after two years of intermittent fasting!

"It took me more years than I could count to struggle with my weight. Finally, I gave up. Nevertheless, when I employed intermittent fasting, everything changed. Since I melted into a petite slender figure and improved my well-being, I felt alive. I gained so much confidence in my youth again. I have trophies to prove that I am not a marathon runner but a 1st place winner. Intermittent fasting helped me to not only budget my food expenses. I saw the big picture of my entire finances and cleaned the house. I now coach women in finances, free up money they did not know was available, and own things they previously could not afford."

3. Post menopause: Sonia West

SONIA'S LIFE was at its worst at 57: she was diagnosed with cancer unexpectedly. Coping with the symptoms was crashing her mental and physical health, and she saw no hope of recovery.

Until she discovered a Facebook group on intermittent fasting, the stories in the group were fascinating. These stories inspired her to implement IF to regain control of her health.

Seven months later, Sonia lost 40 pounds and was mentally and physically in a well-rounded space. She was super impressed with her tight skin that bounced back without flabs and stretch marks. She gained the much-needed confidence and strength to cope with the effects of cancer. But living with cancer was not satisfactory. Sonia engaged in the Daniel fast and prayer in January with her church. She asked the church to pray for her. She kept saying, "As Christ Jesus is, so am I in this world. Jesus has no cancer in His body, and neither do I. I am free from this." In faith, she visited the doctor and was ecstatic to report to her church that her new test report returned negative tumour markers. It was as if they had never existed. Two years later, she is still giving all the glory to YHWH. "I obtained the energy and mental clarity to be creative, set goals and achieve them. For example, I started my own Youtube channel."

The standard tool all these women use is as simple as it can be - fasting for the hours that work best for their schedules. Initially, with a bit of trial and error, the results are all-encompassing and stable.

Intermittent fasting is fasting intermittently, precisely, and not perpetually. First, you fast for a certain decided period. Then, you eliminate snacks and finally eat less often by skipping meals. The longer the fasting hours are, 16 hours, 18 hours, or 22 hours, the better results you will get because IF kicks in autophagy. Autophagy triggers the body's sustainability system to recycle, process, and remove damaged components while generating new cells. As a result, intermittent fasting blesses you with improved body metabolism, weight loss, visceral fat reduction, and reverses type-2 diabetes, cancer, brain and heart-related diseases, and more. Ultimately, IF leads to an extended and healthy lifespan.

2

HORMONE HARMONIZATION & RESURRECTING THE 12 SYSTEMS

Of the major events in a woman's life, going through menopause is one such event. While it may seem like a daunting experience to go through, as someone who has been there and done that, I can truly testify that there is a silver lining.

It truly is a blessing not having to deal with the monthly visitor. Here is some enlightenment on menopause, what it is, why it happens, a delve into hormone fluctuations, and how to deal with them.

The ME-NO-Pause Story

Menopause is a natural, non-medically induced process leading to the permanent end of menstruation. It is a very gradual process that takes place over three stages.

The first stage, known as peri-menopause or "menopause transition," can begin between 45-55 and lasts 7 to 10 years. Gradually your ovaries start to produce less estrogen during this time. Peri-menopause lasts up until menopause, when the ovaries stop releasing eggs permanently.

Often in multiple women's experiences, it is within the last two years of this peri-menopausal period when the drop in estrogen levels accelerates rapidly, and we feel the symptoms typically associated with menopause. Pregnancy is possible; you will still have your menstrual cycles during this time.

The second stage is menopause, when you no longer have menstrual periods. At this point in life, your ovaries will no longer produce eggs, and you will stop manufacturing most of your estrogen. When you have gone without your monthly cycle for 12 months, the diagnosis of having undergone menopause is declared.

The third stage is post-menopause; as the name suggests, this is the period after you haven't had your period for an entire year. During this time, the symptoms that women most commonly associate with menopause, like hot flashes, may improve. Some unlucky buggers might continue to experience menopausal symptoms even a long time after the menopause transition.

Research has shown that post-menopausal women are more prone to heart disease and osteoporosis. Therefore, being generally active, eating healthily, and ingesting supplements for optimal bone health are vital at this stage.

Menopausal Transitions and Expected Developments

Menopausal symptoms hit each woman differently. For example, I experienced frequent hot flashes and constant sleep disruption. Some other typical symptoms you might encounter as you approach menopause are incontinence, vaginal dryness, and decreasing hormone levels, which result in extensive mood swings.

Some physical changes associated with menopause and ageing include fluctuations in weight and subsequent changes in body shape, like a significant weight shift from the hip area to the central tummy area. In addition, your skin could become significantly dryer. Some women have talked about noticing decreased muscle tone and bone density.

Full disclosure: It's no fun. As women, we'll all have to go through it at some point, so the best we can do is to prepare for it.

To be prepared, we must first know what can happen! So, having discussed the various symptoms briefly, let's discuss why they might happen and how to deal with them.

Unfamiliar period patterns

The first thing you observe might be a noticeable change in your period patterns. They could be longer or shorter than usual and not be as regular. Sometimes you might even bleed more or less than average. Even though you expect these changes, if the periods are happening too closely together, resume after no bleeding for a year, or are generally much too abnormal and out of the ordinary, be sure to consult a doctor about your condition to ensure that it's nothing serious. It is always better to avoid the risk.

Hot flashes

Another ordinary symptom women undergoing this transition deal with are hot flashes. Hot flashes can, unfortunately, last for many years, even after menopause. Changes in levels of estrogen most often cause them. A hot flash is a sudden flare of intense heat in particular or all parts of the body. For example, you might be flushed and see red blotches on your face and neck, accompanied by heavy sweating and cold shivers.

Hot flashes, called night sweats, are sometimes stubborn enough to wake you up suddenly in the middle of the night. They last between 10-30 minutes and can happen at all manner of times, multiple times.

Inconvenient incontinence

Another symptom is related to bladder control, in short, incontinence. Incontinence strikes women with the sudden urge to urinate.

It becomes a urine leak when you sneeze, laugh, and exercise. Incontinence could lead to bladder infections, so visit the doctor for treatment.

Sleep issues

Around midlife, some women start having trouble getting a good night's sleep. I have been robbed of my sleep during this stage too many times. You might be unable to sleep when everyone else settles down for the night or even get up at increasingly early and odd hours. Your internal clock might seem out of whack, or the night sweats may interrupt your slumber.

Vaginal health and sexuality

The vagina can also tend to become drier after menopause. Without natural lubrication, sexual intercourse after menopause can be uncomfortable. Additionally, your sex drive may also be affected. You could lose your interest in sex, or you could end up feeling freer and sexier after having ended your monthly menstrual toil. Beware that sexually transmitted diseases are still frank; wearing a condom with your partner would always be the best precaution against unwanted STD-related transmissions.

Mood swings

Women I have talked to about undergoing the arduous ordeal of menopause talk about how they felt significantly moodier and irritable around this transition time. While there has been no scientific inquiry into this, the possible causes could range from bodily stresses due to the transition, hormonal fluctuations, pre-existing mental illnesses like depression, or other external reasons like family changes, for instance, growing children or aging parents. Having a word with your mental health professional or a gynecologist about what you're experiencing would be an excellent resource to lessen your worries and deal with such matters.

Physical changes

Your body shape and distribution will change significantly. For example, your waist could get bigger, lose muscle, and gain more fat. Your skin may get thinner, and your muscles and joints may feel stiff and achy. Some women have also experienced symptoms that include pains, heart palpitations, and headaches. It is difficult to predict how often women will experience menopausal symptoms and their severity, as mainly changing hormone levels cause them. No one shoe fits all.

Hormonal Changes: Harmonization Yields Harmony

Time and time again, you'll hear the terms' hormonal changes' taking the brunt and blame for the symptoms you'll experience during the menopause transition.

So, what are hormones? They are essential for life and health. They tell different body parts what and when to do things. Hormones are chemicals in the human body that help coordinate functions by carrying messages through your bloodstream to your tissues, muscles, organs, and skin.

Various factors and processes can lead to hormone fluctuations. For example, when you undergo menopausal transitions, there is a significant decrease in the body's capacity to produce estrogen. Estrogen is a sex hormone that maintains your overall sexual and reproductive health.

As you age, this hormone secretion is negatively affected, and the endocrine system glands do not operate as skilfully. For this reason, older women are more prone to reduced metabolic rate, disturbed sleep patterns, poor bone density, body fat accumulation, and increased blood glucose. Consequently, they are at increased risk of insomnia, fractures, type-2 diabetes, and cognitive decline. As menopause is an age-induced process, women undergoing it struggle with these problems.

This might seem rather dreary as one of the phenomena humans cannot stop is aging, but a quote comes to mind right now: "The bad news is time flies; The good news is you're the pilot." So, while triptans may help with the occasional migraines, here are some natural and safe ways I have seen work on myself that could help balance your hormones.

Habitudes to Harmonize Your Hormones Like Honey

Intermittent fasting

Intermittent fasting harmonizes hormones, as revealed by various studies. It enhances hormonal balance by boosting metabolism and sleep, energizing, and helping you lose weight.

PROTEIN'S INSULIN Effect

You must consume an abundance of protein every day. Protein provides essential amino acids. Your body can't make them on its own. In addition, protein helps produce peptide hormones, protein-driven hormones. These hormones determine your energy levels, appetite, metabolism, and reproduction.

Furthermore, eating protein stimulates the production of pancreatic peptide YY (PYY), the hormone that makes you feel full while decreasing the hunger hormone ghrelin. Proven in a 3-month study on 156 obese teenagers who consumed high protein breakfast, they increased PYY and amino acids and lost weight due to this satiety.

Consume protein-rich prepared animal food equal to or less than 4 ounces sourced from various meats, fowl, fish, and cheese daily. In addition, vegans and vegetarians may intake daily concentrated protein and carbohydrates equal to or less than 8 ounces from legumes, beans, peas, lentils, nuts, quinoa, and amaranth. Experts recommend that women eat 20–30 grams of protein per meal.

Consuming protein first at mealtime stimulates insulin, suppressing the appetite and, by default, makes us feel satisfied faster so that we only consume what we need. Therefore, eat protein at every meal first to adjust body composition favorably.

Redemptive Exercise

Shocker! Daily exercise is good for you! The amount of physical activity you engage in influences your hormonal health. It improves your blood flow and increases the sensitivity of your hormone receptors, enhancing the delivery of signals and nutrients to various parts of your body.

Regarding aging, physical activity has positively correlated with boosting muscle-maintaining hormones like testosterone, insulin-like growth factor-1 (IGF-1), dehydroepiandrosterone (DHEA), and the human growth hormone (HGH), all of which tend to decline with age.

Exercise also increases insulin sensitivity. Recognize this fantastic yield because insulin, as a hormone, enables your cells to take sugar from your blood and use it for energy. People with high levels of insulin resistance are prone to illnesses like diabetes, obesity, and heart diseases because their cells cannot effectively react to insulin. Physical activities like strength, cardio, and high-intensity interval training reverse insulin resistance. For women who cannot engage in such intense exercise routines for various reasons, taking a daily walk will increase hormone levels and improve their quality of life.

Ideal weight maintenance

Time and time again, an increase in weight is linked to hormonal imbalances and general body disturbance. Weight imbalances lead to later-life complications in insulin sensitivity and interfere with reproductive health. Obesity hampers ovulation causing infertility, and generally adds wear and tear to the bodily systems.

Serendipitously, weight loss aids those suffering from the effects of weight gain. If we're not aiming for skinny, we're aiming for healthy. Eating foods within your calorie range will help maintain a good hormonal balance.

THE STRESS-BREAKING point

Too much stress can wear you out mentally and physically if you don't appropriately deal with it. Your body has cortisol, which helps you cope with long-term stressors. Events that cause stress produce cortisol, and the response typically ends once the pressure is over. However, if your body is under chronic stress, your feedback mechanisms get impaired, and your hormone levels cannot properly return to average balance. High cortisol levels mean ravenous appetite, meaning you'll crave all the fatty high-sugar snacks. You will reap better benefits from cutting these snacks out of your life. Or else they increase your calorie intake and result in eventual obesity. High cortisol levels consistently over the long term affect glucose production from noncarbohydrate sources, leading to increased blood sugar levels which causes insulin resistance.

Making time for activities that you find fun and engaging will surely lower your cortisol levels. Also, you can exercise and listen to relaxing music to soothe yourself. Mind over matter!

CONSUME MORE healthy fats

Not all fats are bad. Instead, including more high-quality natural fats in your daily diet will reduce insulin resistance and appetite. The fats you aim to eat here are medium-chain triglycerides (MCTs), unique fats not stored in fat tissues but taken directly to your liver for energy storage, creating more calorie burning.

Omega-3s are healthy fats that help increase insulin sensitivity by reducing inflammatory markers and overall inflammation. Additionally, omega-3s prevent cortisol levels from growing when people are chronically stressed.

Devour healthy fats from avocados, dry fruits, almonds, walnuts, macadamia nuts, olives, olive oil, coconut oils, and many unrefined foods!

CHECK out the Mediterranean diet

Much research has shown that the Western diet, primarily composed of refined and processed sugars and animal foods, is linked to higher estrogen levels, a breast and ovarian cancer risk factor. The Mediterranean-style diet, on the other hand, is rich in seeds, whole grains, high-fiber foods, legumes, and fish. All these help significantly reduce estrogen levels. Moreover, long-term adherence to this diet has manifestly reduced breast cancer risk during menopause significantly.

Harmonized hormones are equal to well-being. They must be in tip-top shape for your body to function optimally and to the best of its capacity. Remember this. No matter how old you are, even though aging is beyond your control, you will take steps to manage and harmonize your hormones.

Intermittent Fasting Impacts Hormones

ESTROGEN

Estrogen is the collective name of three female hormones – estradiol, released by the ovaries during your reproductive years; estriol, released during pregnancy; and estrone, secreted after menopause. Estrogen, in its healthy levels, develops our sexual characteristics, regulates menstrual cycles, and maintains cholesterol levels.

It protects against cardiovascular disease, prevents inflammation, keeps skin soft and supple, and affects memory. However, when estrogen is imbalanced, it could lead to symptoms similar to PMS, peri-menopause, and menopause. I'm talking about decreased sex drive, irregular periods, weight gain, hair loss, fatigue, brain fog, memory problems, night sweats, etc.

Estrogen regulation through IF

Intermittent fasting helps you maintain the correct estrogen levels. The amount of estrogen is directly proportional to the growth hormone our body produces. But as we grow older, the levels of both estrogen and growth hormones start abating. So as fasting helps increase growth hormone, it helps maintain optimal estrogen levels.

But if your body produces estrogen more profusely, intermittent fasting also resolves that since IF cleans your body at the cellular level, thereby expelling any toxic estrogen from your body.

When your estrogen is balanced, breast cancer is naturally at bay. A study conducted on women receiving treatment for breast cancer concluded that the ones who intermittently fasted observed a 70% reduction in cancer recurrence.

To harmonize estrogen:

1. Have a fiber-rich diet.
2. Stay away from stress.
3. Avoid drinking alcohol.
4. Keep caffeine consumption in check.

Progesterone

Progesterone is an essential female hormone crucial in maintaining your monthly cycles, pregnancy, and embryo formation. It balances estrogen, oversees breast development, regulates body temperature, and stabilizes blood sugar levels. In addition, it has a calming effect on the brain. So, when it is balanced, you feel less anxious and irritated.

. . .

PROGESTERONE REGULATION **through IF**

However, progesterone levels decline naturally during peri-menopause and menopause. They also start dropping when you have a poorly functioning thyroid, intake too much sugar, intake antidepressants and are deficient in vitamins A, B6, and C.

Intermittent fasting supports progesterone, but only if you are being cautious. A fast is only prescribed at certain times during your monthly cycle during peri-menopause, or you can deplete this hormone. For example, I won't recommend fasting five to seven days before and during your menstruation. But if you have achieved menopause, what's to stop you?

Testosterone

Testosterone is a primary sex hormone that triggers sexual desire in women. It maintains muscle mass, keeps you energetic, maintains memory, builds bones, and cares for your well-being. However, like other hormones, this hormone peaks at around 25 and starts falling off. Low testosterone levels make building muscles, controlling blood sugar, and performing other metabolic actions difficult. It also lowers sex drive.

TESTOSTERONE REGULATION **through IF**

Intermittent fasting helps you exercise more control over testosterone. It corrects insulin resistance. So, fasting keeps your insulin levels in check, improving your testosterone levels. In addition, a study concluded that intermittent fasting reduces leptin levels, a hunger hormone. This decrease further triggers an immediate restoration of testosterone.

To increase testosterone:

1. Enhance your protein intake.
2. Learn to manage stress.

3. Have an adequate amount of sunshine to boost your vitamin D levels.
4. Indulge sound sleep.

Thyroid

The thyroid hormone secreted by a beautiful butterfly-shaped gland in front of the windpipe is vital in regulating your body's metabolism. It oversees the functioning of mitochondria, controls your weight, governs the metabolism of carbohydrates, protein, and fat, adjusts body temperature, controls blood flow, regulates vitamin usage, and more.

Any imbalance in the thyroid hormone could interfere with your menstrual cycle. However, more often than not, thyroid imbalances happen during peri-menopause and menopause owing to the ovaries containing thyroid receptors and the thyroid gland having ovary receptors.

Consequently, when you lose estrogen and testosterone during menopause, you may compromise thyroid function. A body that does not produce enough hormones develops hypothyroidism. It is a condition where the immune system attacks the thyroid gland and creates inflammation. On the other hand, greater thyroid levels mean an overactive thyroid, termed hyperthyroidism. It is called Grave's disease, recognized by the abnormal enlargement of the thyroid gland.

The thyroid gland governs how fast the body burns fat; therefore, a sluggish metabolism encourages weight gain. Bolster the vitality of the thyroid by:

- Increasing nutrients that support the thyroid
- Consuming selenium works with other trace minerals found naturally in unrefined foods like whole wheat, brown rice, nuts, and mushrooms.

- Sprouting whole brown rice to reduce the phytic acid, a cleansing constituent. The gamma-oryzanol antioxidant plentiful in rice bran harmonizes the hormones by regulating the pituitary gland and converting fat to lean body mass while strengthening the muscular system.
- Adding shiitake mushrooms to fermented rice bran enhances the immune-boosting value.
- Consuming seaweeds rich in iodine benefits the thyroid, is concentrated in calcium and iron, aids weight loss, and lowers cholesterol and fat in the blood. Hijiki, arame, wakame, kombu and any member of the kelp family. They relieve hormone imbalance that affects the thyroid, benefit the kidneys, soften hard tissues and masses, and build strong bones and teeth.
- Consuming a maximum daily dosage of 1–2 tablespoons or 1–8 grams of sea moss gel or 1000mg capsule with your doctor's permission.
- Supplementing with Vitamin B_{12} combats hypothyroidism.
- Preventing thyroid injury by undertaking low-impact exercises like walking.

Thyroid regulation through IF

Intermittent fasting helps you regulate your thyroid levels. In addition to helping you lose weight, it lowers insulin levels, promotes metabolic flexibility, and reduces inflammation. So, can people who are diagnosed with thyroid disease intermittently fast safely? Various other factors are essential for fasting to work effectively:

1. It would help if you slept adequately.
2. It would help if you dealt with stress actively.
3. It would be best to consume a nutrient-rich whole foods diet.

I recommend speaking to your doctor, but when you adopt healthy lifestyle measures, I see no reason you cannot fast.

MELATONIN

The pineal gland releases the melatonin hormone in the middle of the brain. Melatonin, called the sleep/wake hormone, regulates your internal clock and circadian rhythm. It is produced more during evening darkness as the body prepares to induce deep, healthy sleep. It also affects sex hormones, boosts the immune system, improves mood, stimulates growth hormone production, and decreases cortisol.

Note here that melatonin doesn't work in isolation. It interacts with other hormones and contributes to your overall well-being.

Let's take the example of insulin. Melatonin levels are highest during night-time, while insulin levels are at their lowest because melatonin slows insulin production while you sleep. So, naturally, when you are asleep, your energy needs are less than when you are awake. But what if melatonin levels are low, not suppressing insulin at night? Consequently, your pancreas, which secretes insulin, will not get to rest at night, leading to an anomaly in the long run.

Similarly, melatonin also plays a vital role in defining your menopausal symptoms. During menopause, serotonin levels also fall when estrogen levels sharply decline, and melatonin serum levels gradually decrease. Serotonin is the natural feel-good chemical that makes you feel focused, happy, emotionally stable, and calm.

This wacky relationship between insulin, melatonin, estrogen, and serotonin is enough to wreak havoc during menopause, leading to mood swings and sleep disorders. What's more, melatonin also impacts cortisol levels. Melatonin is high during the night, lowering the production of cortisol and encouraging rest and repair. In the morning, cortisol levels hike, and those of melatonin decline to make you feel energetic. But this cycle doesn't shut down properly if you have chronic stress. Cortisol stays high at night, and melatonin remains insufficient, leading to a lack of sleep.

Improper sleep affects not only your cortisol, insulin, serotonin, and estrogen hormone but also your melatonin hormone. So, if you have insomnia, and sleep disorders, let's fix that.

Melatonin regulation through IF

IF revamps and restores your circadian rhythm, resetting your sleep-wake cycle. Circadian rhythm mainly depends on sunlight, but food is also a time cue. When you fast, you follow set mealtimes, restoring your natural circadian rhythm.

People who fast are also shown to have a higher level of HGH. This hormone boosts the body's functioning while you sleep, repairing your muscles and melting fat.

To further improve your melatonin levels naturally, include these food items in your non-fasting hours:

- A cup of warm milk at bedtime is a natural source of melatonin. Skip this if you are lactose intolerant.
- Nuts like cashews, almonds, and pistachios are also excellent sources of melatonin.
- Consume salmon and tuna, rich in omega-3, magnesium, and vitamin D.
- Goji berries, native to China, are also a natural source of melatonin.
- All kinds of mushrooms are a natural source of melatonin. Please include them in your meals or use them as a topping.
- Corn and brown rice are also helpful in inducing a good night's sleep.
- Bananas, be it a banana shake or eating a whole banana, can help boost melatonin levels.

Like other women in their 50s and over, I struggled with a lack of sleep as I aged because maturing bodies start producing more of some hormones and reduce the production of others; however, as I started my weight loss journey using IF, I realized that IF has also smoothened my sleep cycles and reset my circadian rhythm because IF served a healthier lifestyle that harmonized my hormones naturally.

INSULIN

I cannot stress how insulin is crucial for maintaining blood sugar levels, cell growth and repair, brain function, and weight control.

The purpose of the insulin hormone is to regulate blood sugar levels in the body. If you have diabetes, it depicts that your insulin hormone is imbalanced. Therefore, high insulin levels result in weight gain.

When you eat, the food breaks down to release energy. Carbohydrates in the food break down into glucose. After digestion, glucose enters the bloodstream, and its levels temporarily rise. The pancreas then secretes insulin to move the glucose from the blood into cells. The pancreas must release more insulin to address the increased glucose in the blood. Insulin unlocks the way glucose enters the bloodstream.

However, with consistently elevated insulin levels, you risk developing insulin resistance. This condition happens when cells become accustomed to the overabundant presence of insulin, not allowing the free flow of glucose from the bloodstream to cells. Chronic stress is another condition in which insulin levels stay elevated. Perpetually elevated insulin levels cripple your body's metabolism.

INSULIN REGULATION through IF

Insulin can make you fat no matter how cautious you are. If you are secreting high insulin levels, it will make you fat.

DOES that mean diabetic people who take insulin are inclined to get fat? Yes, to an extent. However, if you are pre-diabetic, you can reverse the issue. Pre-diabetic people, i.e., those more likely to get diabetes in the coming decade, can prevent themselves from entering this vicious circle by revamping their diet and engaging IF to intercept insulin resistance and step back from the trap.

Natural treatments against pre-diabetic symptoms:

- Lose your extra pounds to diminish the chances of developing diabetes. Increased physical activity and dietary changes can curtail the 58% risk of contracting diabetes.
- Follow a diabetic food plan that includes fiber and protein-rich foods like sprouts, flaxseeds, quinoa, chia seeds, wild salmon, and grass-fed beef.
- Increase chromium in your diet by increasing the intake of nuts, eggs, grapes, and whole grains.
- Keep a check on magnesium intake. Take magnesium supplements or include magnesium-rich foods, like legumes, nuts, seeds, and leafy vegetables.
- The best way to naturally reverse diabetes is by incorporating Ceylon cinnamon into your diet. Add a pinch or stick to your hot chocolate, tea, and curries.
- CoQ10 supplements can also prevent pre-diabetes. It's known to lower plasma glucose and hemoglobin A1C levels.
- The last essential supplement is ginseng. It is known to reduce blood sugar levels and control insulin levels.

Insulin imbalance causes symptoms of obesity, delayed periods, frequent urination, fatigue, and more.

That's where IF will rescue you. If you eat constantly, your body's insulin levels remain high. However, when you fast for a certain number of hours, your body's insulin levels fall, obliging your body's cells to be more sensitive to insulin. Fortunately, this also leads to rapid fat melting.

. . .

Cortisol

When your body is stressed, the adrenal gland produces and secretes a hormone called cortisol. Cortisol works by freeing up blood sugar to provide enough energy to the body to defend itself from any stress and pressure. Cortisol also boosts your blood pressure to supply enough oxygen and nutrients through the body.

When the body returns to its normal state, cortisol levels lower. However, the sympathetic nervous system goes into overdrive when you are under chronic stress. High cortisol levels facilitate high stress, high blood pressure, poor immune system, digestive disorders, and vulnerability to autoimmune diseases. Any imbalance in the cortisol hormone also directly affects your night's sleep.

Cortisol regulation through IF

Cortisol hormone also makes you fat. High cortisol increases glucose levels, thereby increasing insulin and your weight coincidentally.

Your elevated cortisol levels could result from high-stress levels and poor sleep patterns. Here are six quick and natural ways to lower them:

- Stay away from packaged foods, sugary drinks, and refined grain products.
- Skip drinking caffeine and alcohol.
- Consume more whole foods like flaxseeds, fiber-rich fruits, vegetables, oats, beetroot etc.
- Reduce stress levels through deep breathing and doing tasks that reduce anxiety, such as gardening, nature walks, and running barefoot.
- Exercise regularly at your own pace. It doesn't have to be too vigorous, but walking and Zumba dancing work well.
- Take herbs that lower cortisol levels, like ashwagandha, basil leaves, licorice root, and mushrooms like reishi and shiitake.

Intermittent fasting is considered a hormetic stressor. It is a beneficial type of stress that prepares your body to fight against more substantial stressors in the future. However, if you are under too much pressure, I suggest you undertake intermittent fasting by planning to eat three healthy satiating meals per day in an 8-to-10-hour period. Do not overdo fasting because adding more stress may elevate cortisol levels instead of lowering them.

Balanced cortisol enables you to respond to stress and danger, cultivating healthy blood pressure and immune system.

Oxytocin

Oxytocin, the 'love hormone' and 'cuddle chemical,' plays a crucial part in love, increased sexual desire, mother-child bonding, and building connection and trust in relationships. Responses to touch, sexual activity, childbirth, breastfeeding, and the activation of sensory nerves during labour trigger oxytocin.

The hypothalamus gland produces it, and the pituitary gland releases it into the bloodstream and secretes it into the ovaries, brain, uterus, and placenta. However, oxytocin levels fluctuate during menses. It peaks around the time of ovulation. It then decreases during the latter half of the cycle.

Oxytocin has an interesting relationship with other hormones. It makes cells more insulin-sensitive, boosting metabolic flexibility. It also reduces cortisol levels, helping you manage stress levels. Low on sexual desire? Blame the low oxytocin hormone your body produces.

When oxytocin gets imbalanced, you feel little to no pleasure in sex, have difficulty feeling attached in relationships, and it can also lead to long-term depression and anxiety.

Oxytocin regulation through IF

IF and oxytocin are relational. Higher oxytocin levels help you fast more easily and for longer periods. Therefore, when you fast, I recommend connecting with others more intimately. Well, you now have a reason to hug and kiss your partner. *wink*

Natural oxytocin boosters to attain greater well-being:

- Simply smiling.
- Strike your power pose.
- Give a loved one a massage.
- Cuddling or hugging a loved one.
- Exercising only 5 minutes of high-intensity workouts will give you a jump in salivary oxytocin levels.
- Take an outdoor walk.
- Consume your Vitamin C from bell peppers, broccoli, cauliflower, citrus fruits, and tomatoes.
- Capture some sunshine into your eyes and skin.
- Skip the alcohol.
- Listen to your uplifting playlist.
- Add some bonding to your music endeavors by singing or playing a musical instrument in a group.

Leptin

Do you know what regulates your blood pressure and heart rate, controls your metabolism and energy homeostasis, helps regulate the synthesis of your thyroid hormones, decreases glucose-stimulated insulin resistance, and modulates the menstrual cycle? Is it better that with so many hormones in our body, there could also be a weight control hormone? There is indeed one.

I am talking about the star performers of IF - Leptin.

When it works appropriately, it regulates your appetite, suppresses hunger, and prevents you from overeating. A signal from the fat cell to the hypothalamus tells the brain that we have enough nutrition and food. The fat and intestinal cells make it and release it in the white blood cells, ovaries, skeletal muscles, and the lower part of the stomach.

Chronically high levels of leptin over long periods cause leptin resistance. The receptor cells become desensitized, and the body no longer absorbs the hormone. Blocked receptors prevent the feedback loops from returning to the fat cells, driving the fat cells to make more leptin perpetually. Are you always hungry and greedy? That is due to a condition where the abundance of leptin is not working, and your brain never gets the signal, 'I am full.' The symptoms of leptin deficiency are hunger, starvation, and excess.

Another purpose of leptin is to suppress the immune system to calm inflammation. Without enough leptin, women develop higher risks of an autoimmune problem because of the presence of excess inflammation, which weakens the immune system.

Leptin regulation through IF

Engaging IF over time solves leptin resistance, supports a healthy and improved immune system, and suppresses inflammatory conditions. The imbalance in leptin hormone can imbalance your insulin hormone, which throws everything down the drain.

To prevent this, here are some ways to boost leptin:

- Switch to oils like extra virgin olive, avocado, coconut, and ghee. Ghee, in particular, benefits menopause and stimulates leptin.
- Add more greens and colors to your palate.
- Berries like strawberries, blueberries, and cranberries will kick leptin into gear.
- Eat raw, steamed, or roasted vegetables.
- Fish, lean meat, and animal protein also keep leptin balanced.
- Add fibrous foods to your diet, like dark green leafy vegetables, oatmeal, whole grain, legumes, and sprouts.
- Switch to brown rice and other whole grains; abstain from refined ones.

Intermittent Fasting Harmonizes These Hormones

Estrogen, progesterone, testosterone, thyroid, melatonin, serotonin, cortisol, oxytocin, and leptin are all critical hormones in the body. Any imbalance in these hormones would induce high-stress levels and push you to consume abnormally high amounts of sugar.

Intermittent fasters see a drop in insulin resistance and a significant plunge in the biomarkers of oxidative stress. By shortening the eating window, intermittent fasting makes women naturally cut calories and eat less. The resulting weight loss alone enables better sleep. However, intermittent fasting also improves the circadian rhythm and sleep quality because of the satiating foods consumed within the specific eating window that closes three hours before bedtime. This deliberate behavior improves sleep automatically. A well-slept woman is a happier, generous woman ready to move more and capable of managing stress.

So, focus on what you can control - when and what you eat during your eating window. Satisfy and curb your hunger with healthy saturated and monounsaturated fats, whole grains, vegetables, and proteins. Avoid sugar, fructose, refined flour, and vegetable seed oils.

While it is wise for all women to take breaks from intermittent fasting, women at the peri-menopause stage must refrain from fasting close to and during menstruation because hormones control the menstruation cycle. Hormone levels are more stable during postmenopause. When done correctly, intermittent fasting improves insulin responses, lipid levels, blood pressure, and body composition.

Conduct regular hormone checks at all stages to ensure you support healthy hormones during intermittent fasting and make suitable adjustments.

Intermittent fasting causes these hormones to harmonize, and you will soon start living up.

Intermittent Fasting Resurrects the 12 Systems

We all want results, and when I say intermittent fasting gets those results, I mean it. With so many benefits, this form of time-restricted eating has recently gained much attention due to its efficient approach to weight loss and other potential long-term health benefits. At this juncture, I shall briefly touch upon how intermittent fasting positively affects the various systems of your body:

1. Endocrine system

Comprising of a complex network of glands and organs, the integral parts of the endocrine system are the hypothalamus, pineal gland, pituitary gland, thyroid and parathyroid, thymus, adrenal gland, pancreas, and ovary. It is a messenger system that regulates the organs by releasing hormones into the bloodstream through the circulatory system on a feedback loop. These hormones command and coordinate functions in the body. Intermittent fasting ensures these functions: proper sleep, sex, reproduction, growth and development, metabolism, blood pressure, energy level and physical response to injury, emotional response to stress, and mood. In addition, the positive results of intermittent fasting on the endocrine systems present overwhelming metabolic improvements in cardiac and brain function, blood glucose levels, calmness, and weight loss.

2. Cardiovascular system

Intermittent fasting limits many risk factors for the development and occurrence of cardiovascular diseases. The beneficial effect also includes the prevention of hypertension and a positive impact on obese and diabetic patients. Intermittent fasting decreases body weight due to a reduced amount of food consumed. It further has a positive effect on glucose metabolism and increases the sensitivity of tissues, making your cells more responsive to insulin, thereby reducing the risks of diseases like diabetes. It does so by expanding the beta cells of the pancreatic islets. It also limits cardiac hypertrophy.

3. Neurological system

Clinical studies have shown the benefits of IF for epilepsy, multiple sclerosis, and Alzheimer's and for reducing other disease symptoms. The findings from animal studies also show a positive effect of IF on Parkinson's disease, autism spectrum disorder, ischemic stroke, and mood and anxiety disorders. So, adding frequent exercise, limiting calorie intake, and generally being more present will reprogram the Grim Reaper Clock™ and give you some more legroom in this plane called life.

4. Pulmonary system

Intermittent fasting can help with pulmonary system problems like pulmonary arterial hypertension (PAH). It is a rare disease that affects the working of the lungs' arteries and the heart's right side. In other words, it is a disease that increases blood pressure in the lungs' arteries, making it hard to breathe. Research has shown that IF directly enhances right ventricular (RV) function and restructures the gut microbiome. It is a non-pharmacological approach to combat RV dysfunction caused by PAH.

5. Gastrointestinal system

Fasting gives the digestive system a break. It balances gut bacteria, promotes probiotics, and enhances bacterial diversity. Studies show that even short-term fasts could induce long-term benefits to gut health.

6. Dermatological system

IF also significantly affects your skin's appearance because IF triggers autophagy - the "self-cleaning" process that eradicates old, damaged cells and proteins and makes way for new, healthy ones. This process accomplishes glowing skin.

7. Psychological system

Your mental health is equally essential to your physical health, and intermittent fasting delivers benefits here too. When you fast, naturally, your body has fewer toxic materials due to the process of autophagy, making it easier for you to think. In addition, while fasting, the energy you'd usually use to digest food becomes available for brain function.

IF also increases the levels of a brain-derived neurotrophic factor (BDNF) protein in the brain. Low levels of BDNF appear in depression, anxiety, and major depressive disorder. The lower the levels, the more severe the symptoms. IF increases this neuroprotective substance's resistance to damage and encourages the growth of new neurons.

8. Immune system

Intermittent fasting reboots your immune system, regenerates white blood cells for better immune response, and replenishes lost blood cells.

Short-term fasting, like intermittent fasting, urges the body to produce white blood cells to overcome the mild stress of fasting. This process acts as a reboot button for your immune system. It implements disease-fighting cells during the fasting period, rejuvenating the immune system.

9. The reproductive system of women in their 50s and over

"Your eggs have almost reached the dormant stage. You cannot get pregnant." "It gets challenging to get pregnant over the 40s, not to talk about the 50s," are statements women hear from their 20s. But you are 50 and pregnant. How did that happen? Well, because you have a healthy uterus.

"Being naturally pregnant at 50, being a first-time mum without even trying, was a shock and took quite a bit to get used to", says Veronica Lewis, who defied all odds and saw two red lines on a pregnancy test.

Eating healthy makes an appreciable difference, especially with intermittent fasting. This combination helped women overcome polycystic ovary syndrome (PCOS), dysmenorrhea, and infertility. However, one of the research quotes, "Fasting does not appear to have any effect on other reproductive hormones such as estrogen, gonadotropins, and prolactin." Further investigation is required to refute these allegations.

10. Renal system

Studies found that careful fasting, like intermittent fasting, reduces the albumin in the urine. It is a protein made by the liver. A sign of kidney disease is too much albumin in the urine. Moreover, a healthy kidney won't let albumin pass from the blood into the urine. So intermittent fasting indeed has a positive bearing on the renal system.

11. Hematological system

The hematological system consists of blood, bone marrow, and platelets. Short-term fasting, like IF, proved beneficial in adenosine triphosphate (ATP) generation - the molecule that carries energy in the cell, boosts oxygen transportation in red blood cells (RBCs) and promotes erythropoiesis – the production of RBCs. Reduction in RBC in adults can lead to severe conditions like anemia, leukemia, myelodysplastic syndrome, cardiovascular diseases, cognizant impairment, and many more. Engaging IF improves RBC production and function.

. . .

12. Musculoskeletal system

While intermittent fasting increases HGH for building muscles, integrating IF with exercise has helped women in their 50s and older burn fat and build more muscle.

Weight training and resistance training help maintain muscle and melt fat.

But I would like to flash a disclaimer. IF works, but the visibility of results depends on your overall lifestyle and body. So, hold on, ladies, and you will get there!

Let's look at breast cancer and its connection to IF.

Pre- And Post-Menopausal Women with Breast Cancers

Are post-menopausal women more likely to have breast cancer? While this may be true to an extent, various risk factors determine so. Such risk factors include family history, genetic factors, dense breast tissues, personal history of breast cancer, use of birth control pills, alcohol, obesity, induced abortion, lack of pregnancy, pregnancy at a late age, and hormone therapy after menopause.

Just the phase of menopause, pre-menopause, or post-menopause does not cause breast cancer. However, the risk of getting breast cancer increases as women age. Research says that women who achieve menopause after age 55 are at an increased risk of ovarian, uterine, or/and breast cancer. In addition, girls who began menstruating before age 12 are also at a greater risk. The underlying reason is that the longer women are exposed to estrogen, the greater the chances.

The research quotes, "Risk of developing breast cancer increased in both pre-and post-menopausal patients who had early onset of menarche and late menopause possibly due to the increase in the duration of hormonal exposure."

In short, both the peri-menopause and post-menopause phases result in hormone irregularities. Therefore, IF can correct hormonal imbalances, and women can further reduce the risk of breast cancer in pre-menopause and post-menopause. To support the statement, a study on "prolonged nightly fasting and breast cancer prognosis" concludes that extending the nightly fasting intervals is a non-pharmacological strategy to reduce breast cancer recurrence. The same study also mentions that not only what we eat matters, but the time we eat also influences metabolism and cancer. For example, many types of intermittent fasting positively affect cancer outcomes.

I keep talking about hormone imbalance. Next, I will reveal how you can balance hormones naturally.

Harmonize Hormones Naturally

All of this comes down to balancing hormones. So how can you balance your hormones to reduce the chances of breast cancer and keep all your systems working synchronously? Great news, you can do it naturally.

SWITCH to healthy fats

Healthy fats are known for harmonizing hormones. They also act as anti-inflammatory and metabolism boosters.

Some easy to accommodate healthy fat foods include coconut oil, avocado, wild-caught salmon, and grass-fed butter. All of these can be introduced in an IF formula flexibly.

NECESSARY SUPPLEMENTS

No matter how healthily you eat, some nutritional voids still lead to hormonal imbalance. For this, it is necessary to take the required supplements. The essential supplements include:

- Primrose oil for supporting hormonal function. Also, beneficial for polycystic ovary syndrome (PCOS) symptoms and premenstrual syndrome (PMS).

- Vitamin D is another supplement that keeps hormonal imbalances in check.
- Consume bone broth as it aids easy digestion and improves overall health.
- Probiotics for a healthy gut and to eliminate inflammatory diseases like IBD and IBS.
- Adaptogen herbs like ashwagandha for improving overactive thyroid function, cholesterol, blood sugar levels, and other hormonal imbalances. Tulsi and basil leaves are also essential herbs in regulating hormonal imbalance.

Use essential oils

Using carrier oils like coconut oil and shea butter is one way to balance your hormones naturally. In addition, these oils tend to remove toxins from the body. Some recommended essential oils free from chemicals include:

- Clary sage oil: massage five drops of clary sage mixed with coconut oil over the stomach. Doing so reduces the chances of ovarian cancer and uterine cancer in older women.
- Fennel seeds: as you age, gut health and thyroid problems come tumbling down one over another. Consuming fennel seed tea boosts metabolism and digestion and controls thyroid levels. One can also rub a few drops of fennel seed oil over the stomach to correct hormonal imbalance.
- Lavender oil: mix a few drops in your bath water or rub 2 to 3 drops over your temple, wrists, or neck is also known to keep hormones in check.
- Sandalwood oil: apply sandalwood oil over the wrists and bottom of the feet to keep stress at bay.

KEEP check of medications

Ingesting depression medication and birth control pills that include dopamine agonists, corticosteroids, statins, and rexinoids are known to disturb the hormonal imbalance.

Pre-menopausal and post-menopausal women should check the medications they are taking. Intermittent fasting gradually eliminates the need to take medicines in the first place.

SLEEP, sleep, sleep

Getting enough sleep of 7 to 9 hours is the most convenient way to keep hormones balanced. Sleeping keeps the stress hormones, i.e., high cortisol levels, at bay. High cortisol levels are directly linked with high stress, negatively impacting your sleep cycle and disturbing hormonal function.

Where viable, go to bed at least by ten and stick to a regular sleep cycle to treat your hormonal imbalance naturally. It is that easy.

HORMONES ARE critical in stabilizing our body processes. Living a holistic lifestyle integrating intermittent fasting streamlines hormones to a greater extent. Intermittent fasting harmonizes the hormones like honey, regulates the 12 body systems and improves the circadian rhythm.

So, all set? Intermittent fasting is promising, didn't I say? So, let's take another step on this journey. Let me help you break all the barriers.

3

BREAKING THROUGH THE BARRIERS

Was Rome built in a day? As you venture on to your intermittent fasting journey initially, understand that getting into the groove and making your body move is not be an overnight project. It may take a reasonable amount of time to get used to your new lifestyle but expect great results.

As of now, you're making good progress! Being with me and getting this far into it means you're willing to put effort and some natural elbow grease into this endeavor. That is step one.

So now you know the various benefits of intermittent fasting, and it's good that you want to start a.s.a.p. and strive to live your healthiest life. But how do you go about it? Stay with me, and I will talk about things you must keep in mind while preparing your body for intermittent fasting and how you will adjust to it eventually.

There are several types and ranges of intermittent fasting methods that you can pick up, and the style you choose is ultimately up to you.

Preparation for a Successful Fast

First, you need a solid base for the IF method to accelerate weight loss and optimal health.

For instance, you will reap the desired results from intermittent fasting if you plan for good sleep quality, manage stress properly, manage your relationships with others appropriately, exercise regularly, and have found significant spiritual fulfillment. Let us now look at some practical steps you can take to prepare for a successful fast:

Reimaging

If you aim for nothing, you hit nothing. So it's always good when you can visualize realistic goals for yourself. Rather than hoping for any vague change, setting attainable goals and writing them down to solidify them would do a world of good. I often find myself more willing to undertake activities when I know there is a solid outcome at the end of it.

With intermittent fasting, you can expect results if you work smart at sticking to it, but this sticking to it part can be challenging. First, you need to know why you're doing what you're doing. So, when you are at a point in the fast when things are getting tough and giving up feels like the best option, look at the goals you had written down for yourself and the significant purpose you were working towards when you initiated this goal.

Work to manifest your written words. Be it to lose weight for an ex's wedding two months away or improve your gut health? Any motivation is good if it gets you moving. So start the morning with a glass of water and your personalized motto, 'I sleep like a baby, eliminate the clutter around me and engage in fun activities.'

Reality Check - Current Routine Evaluation

Sit down for a good twenty-one minutes and evaluate your daily life patterns. What needs fixing? Use this time to make decisions purposely, how you plan to achieve them and stick to the plan to get to the best standard possible. You could look at the following dimensions and see how you can improve them:

- Sleep hygiene
- Manage stress
- Relationships
- Eating quality
- Exercise regime
- Spiritual fulfilment

Sleep Hygiene

Good sleep is the cornerstone of a good day and a healthy life. This seemingly inconsequential daily activity that we participate in is crucial for our overall well-being. As already discussed, long-term overexposure to cortisol and other stress hormones will disrupt almost all your body's processes and disastrously affect your health.

Your body has an internal clock that enters a period of sleep followed by a period of wake time every 24 hours, and this cycle roughly coincides with the 24-hour night-time-daytime cycle. The production of cortisol also follows a roughly similar process which drops to its lowest levels at around midnight and peaks right after you wake up.

Studies have shown that insomnia and sleep deprivation cause your body to secrete more cortisol to stimulate daytime alertness. Therefore, a good night's sleep is vital for balancing cortisol levels. In addition, your body needs regular restful sleep to stay healthy and function properly. You may have heard that adults need 7-9 hours of sleep to stay healthy and function properly.

Getting a good night's sleep might be more challenging as you age. About 50% of older adults have reported insomnia, difficulty sleeping, early awakening, or tiredness on waking. Your sleep patterns could change, and you could be experiencing shorter sleep duration, disturbed sleep at night, and increased nocturnal awakenings, or on the inverse, you could sleep excessively. On the other hand, taking an afternoon or day nap might have become part of your daily norm. These unrestful sleep patterns could be for reasons like a shift in insulin, melatonin, or other hormone levels or a change in circadian rhythm, the natural, internal process that regulates one's sleep-wake cycle. While these changes may naturally occur with age, this doesn't mean they are not bad for you and should just be accepted.

Indulging a good night's sleep may seem challenging, but it is in no way impossible. Take the following steps to improvement:

Lower the thermostat

Have you ever wondered why getting out of the covers in winter can be so daunting? Other than the fact that the outside world is cold and dreary, your desire to sleep longer is because a cold room temperature often encourages you to want to curl up under the covers. Cooler temperature accelerates falling asleep, and you get drowsy easier in this cocoon of warmth inside your blanket, which creates a warm "microclimate" around the body, making you want to sleep more. Set your thermostat between 18° 20°C or 65°-68°F. You're going to find yourself sound asleep.

Take a warm shower or bath

To make yourself fall asleep faster, ease into a hot bath. It can trigger temperature changes in your body, promoting relaxation and sleepiness. In addition, studies have shown that people who routinely take warm baths and showers within 2 hours before bedtime report better sleep quality.

Keep your electronics away for half an hour before going to bed

The blue light emitted by your phone and smart device's screen is horrible for anybody hoping to fall asleep quickly. Exposure to bright or blue light within two hours of bedtime causes people to stay alert longer and feel sleepy later because the blue light restrains melatonin production. This hormone controls your sleep-wake cycle.

Exercise earlier in the day

Research has shown that people who often struggle to fall asleep or get a restful sleep at night tend to have trouble lowering their internal core temperature when settling down to sleep. Therefore, exercising and implementing any workout routine during the daytime can help better regulate your body temperature. However, it would be best if you made it a point to workout at least 4 hours away from bedtime, especially in a brightly lit gym, as it could be counterproductive and interfere with women with sleep disorders.

Add meditation to your day

Several studies have shown that certain practices, including prayerful meditation, help promote better sleep. First, meditate at home by choosing a place free from distractions where you can sit quietly and not be disturbed. Begin by breathing slowly. As you breathe, focus on a personalized phrase of your choice and repeat it to maintain relevance without losing focus. Personally, imagining that the Creator and Possessor of Heaven and Earth cuddling me brings me unspeakable joy. So, I inhale the euphoric air of Heaven, and I repeat, "You satisfy me with good things." On this note, I appreciate the beautiful blessings I consistently receive. "Your presence satisfies me more than the richest of foods." "You are such a blanket of pleasure to my soul." My method for memorizing the Scriptures.

Breathe Easy

In addition, practice this 4-7-8 breathing method. It involves the following steps:

- Sit straight and place your tongue's end directly behind your top front teeth.
- Breathe in and out through your mouth while verbalizing the word 'woosh.'
- Take a second and slowly inhale through your nose to the count of four.
- Hold your breath and count to 7.
- Then, exhale through your mouth again, and this time count to 8 while verbalizing the word 'woosh.'

Do the above steps three times in a row. However, doing it twice daily to oxygenate your body yields the best results.

CREATE a bedtime routine

By creating a bedtime routine and keeping a consistent sleep schedule, you are allowing yourself to set your internal clock in an organized manner. For example, an inconsistent slumber time may confuse your internal clock with random cues. In reverse, suppose you routinely and consistently expose yourself to the same patterns of light and dark day in and day out. In that case, your body soon gets accustomed to it, which can help you reset your internal clock to the appropriate socially acceptable sleep and wake-up time. For example, you could start bedtime routines by settling down at a particular time daily, relaxing your body, writing in your journal, listening to a relaxing playlist before sleeping, and reading a book. For instance, instead of watching TV, I spend time in grateful reflection, writing in my journal while listening to a relaxing playlist.

DISCLAIMER: *If nothing seems to work, believe me, IF will. I have tried and tested this time and again that IF does make you sleep better.*

Stress Mitigation

The first step to managing stress is identifying what is stressing you. It could be a work-related issue, or it could even be a personal relationship-related issue. Once you have determined what is stressing you out, you can work towards solving or dealing with this stressor.

One stressor I have struggled with, and I'm sure many older people with extensive networks grapple with, is unresolved fights and problems with people around them. I wouldn't say I'm a person who holds many grudges, but when I do, I hold on for far longer than necessary, which benefits nobody.

Long-term, unresolved anger connects to health conditions such as high blood pressure, depression, anxiety, and heart disease. Plus, unforgiveness is the channel to cancer. In such cases, practicing forgiveness and learning to let go would do wonders to lower your stress levels.

Thank you to those who so skillfully manipulated, tortured, and caused me pain. I choose to love them and let God judge them. I am so grateful to Holy Spirit for closing those doors. I forget all the wrong things, cast all my cares on Him, and receive His help and divine council. He is God on the throne. He sees and knows everything. I gave it all to Jesus Christ, who strengthened me. God gets the glory out of my pain, wounds, and infirmities. He is using my bruises and attack wounds to elevate me. It is Christ Jesus who fights for me, honors and promotes me. My trust in Jesus and our vision and goals drive my green present and clear, bright future. I chose to think about the beautiful, excellent things and the loving-kindness of God throughout my life. He is a good God and works all these things for my good. The hand of the LORD is on me, blessing me 100-fold. Thank You, El Shaddai.

Other than this, you can come across several different sorts of stressors. Below are some highly effective strategies to reduce stress in your daily life.

. . .

LISTEN to music

Make yourself a playlist of songs that soothe and calm you. When you're feeling overwhelmed and stressed, pop on your head/earphones and submerge into some tunes. Studies have shown that playing calm and soothing music positively affects the brain and body. Not only does it help lower blood pressure, but it can also reduce your cortisol levels.

TALK about your issues with a friend

Catharsis always works for me. Prayer is my first option. A good ranting session will lower those cortisol levels right away. Talking with a friend will help you relieve stress and significantly make your stressor easier and more bearable. If you cannot eliminate it because it is your ex or boss, ...

TALK yourself through it

Sometimes life happens, and talking to a friend is not possible. In such cases, give yourself some time and talk it out loud! Or writing your problems/stressors out can help. If you don't want people to think you're a bit coo-coo, consider isolating yourself and giving yourself a pep talk – start by telling yourself why you're stressed out, then list what you need to do and how you will go about doing it. And lastly, tell yourself everything will be okay.

EAT RIGHT!

You can never underestimate the power of food and how greatly it contributes to your quality of life. Having a proper diet and one's stress levels are very closely related. When a person is overwhelmed, eating is often the last thing on their mind. And if they do want to eat, it's often fatty snack foods that they reach out to as a pick-me-up. So, avoid the sugars and pick up fruit the next time you crave something sweet. Eating fish that have high omega-3 fatty acids and fresh vegetables are excellent ways, in the long term, to keep your body healthy and reduce the symptoms of stress. Furthermore, stress eaters tend to cut and swallow. Tip: intuitively chew your food 47 times.

Drink tea

Instead of getting your daily dose of coffee or chugging down energy drinks, sip green tea. Not only does it contain healthy antioxidants and theanine, but it also has less caffeine than coffee and amino acids that almost instantly calm your nerves. Soothing nerves with a relaxing cup of tea is how you'll find me beating the stress in my life.

Breath in and out

Apostle Paul, in Acts 17:25, knew what was up when he said that God gave all mankind life, breath and everything. While "taking a deep breath" may seem like clichéd advice, it holds very true regarding stress. Deep breathing works by oxygenating your blood, grounding your body, and clearing your mind.

Sleep well!

Utilizing the previous tips and tricks, get a good night's sleep, as lack of sleep can stress a person out immensely. An excellent restful sleep session of 7-9 hours can be a very effective stress buster.

I know I keep repeating the importance of sleep, but take my word for it -- sleeping is heavenly.

Synergistic Relationships

Toxic relationships happen, and that's life. The best you can do for yourself is identify the people who make you feel bad or are messing with your life and work to resolve your issues. Suppose saying goodbye is not an option or cutting them out. Cold-hearted as the second option may be, you must take some necessary actions to live a long, happy, stress-free life.

Even the Proverbs cautions us to choose our friends wisely in Proverbs 12:26, 18:24, 22:24-25 & 27:6. I have already reaped the consequences of having too many friends chosen indiscriminately. Now that I know that my friends help determine who I become, I am actively choosing excellent examples who inspire me to copy their excellence.

Giving antagonists your time and energy is unsuitable for both of you. How to identify these people and their toxic behaviors? Red flags:

- Chronic anger
- Chronic sarcasm
- Disparaging humor
- Having a punitive mindset
- Excessive insecurity
- Exhibiting excessively manipulative behavior
- Predominate self-centeredness!

If you associate with people with these traits, run in the opposite direction when possible. Better save yourself the future headache and heartache that toxic relationships bring. You can't eliminate them that easily, like in a workplace or family setting. Work to set boundaries!

Eating Quality

Mind over matter. That's how you approach things when it comes to food. Look at the goals you wrote down for yourself and ask yourself why you are embarking on this intermittent fasting journey before taking that 'much-deserved cheat day.' We all know the only person you're cheating on is yourself. So, write down the following in your journal:

'I take authority over my appetite. I dominate food; food does not control me. I overthrow all the addictions to sugar, milk, cheese, and ice cream.' Be sure to write down the names of the food you find particularly hard to resist. Also, write down the "Why" like 'It makes me feel bloated, look pregnant, causes inflammation, itching' etc. Then note what you will accomplish.

Food is not illicit, unlike many other addictive substances, which makes overcoming it so much more complex but not impossible. Instead, overcoming food addiction and mastering how to eat for strength involves keeping in mind the following things:

- Learning how food functions in your body, what it takes to eat in a nutritious way, and what it means to overeat while punishing with food consistently will help develop a more beneficial relationship with food.
- Take stock of your eating habits. Sometimes people use food to alleviate stress, while food might be a source of punishment for others who eat to the point of feeling ill or ashamed. Anxiety and stressors drive food addiction. Taking stock of these behaviors and biases will help break down the most likely triggers of indulging in food addiction and can help unearth some of the reasons behind the addiction. Before opening the fridge or reaching for the food, ask yourself why you want this.
- Learning about your likes and dislikes, strengths and weaknesses, and pain and pleasure can help you move away from addiction because it can ease some of the uncertainty that you are using food to build walls to protect.

Exercise Regime

Movement and getting your blood moving release endorphins that instantly lift your mood. When I say exercise, I don't mean only powerlifting at the gym or training for a marathon. Taking a short, sweet walk around the office or standing up from your desk and taking a long stretch offers a good sense of relief and alleviates some stress. I will discuss this further.

Spiritual Fulfillment

We are humans made in God's image and His likeness. To not know our Creator and the purpose for which He put us on earth would render our existence, frankly speaking, meaningless. Only with a deeper understanding of God first and ourselves second can we attain true satisfaction. As much as I go on about physical health and the importance of a wholesome, earthy substance, fulfillment comes from our daily spiritual sustenance from our LORD and Savior. For holistic healing, we must also tend to the spirit's wounds.

I am the daughter of El Shaddai, the Most High God. I consult and obey my manufacturer's guide and act according to Joshua 1:8-9 and Psalm 1:1-3, my strategy for success and prosperity. I live by His Spirit within me and travel in the slipstream of the Kingdom of Heaven. In John 5:6, Christ Jesus asked, "Will you be made whole?" Naomi exclaimed, "Absolutely, yes, yes, yes, Master! And so it is, as Proverbs 4:20-22 agrees that the Word of God is healing to all my flesh.

In Daniel 11:32, Prophet Daniel wrote that the spiritually mature people who know their God display strength and do exploits. My Father appreciates my fasting and makes me an oasis in a dry and thirsty land. Therefore, I trust Him and depend solely on El Shaddai, who rewards me with Deuteronomy 28:1-14 blessings and all the blessings of Abraham, Isaac, Jacob, and Israel.

I know that I am loved, and I cuddle Father tightly in love. He confers the benefits of Psalm 91:14-16 on me. And all Grace abounds towards me because God is for me. I am His favorite child. His revelation makes it easy for me to focus and meditate on things that are true, noble, just, pure, lovely, and good reports. So, I choose to reverence YHWH and keep His commandments, making me a whole woman. Ecclesiastes 12:13-14.

We become like the God we worship, and we all worship someone or something, whether we worship ourselves or our intellect. Where are you spiritually? Do you know who you are? Your spirituality dictates your identity. Once you know who you are, you will recognize what you truly want and where you are going, and achieve your destiny. So, enjoy the journey of your discovery.

Visual Inspiration

Keeping track requires assessing how intermittent fasting is perfect for you and illustrating your progress. It tracks what's working for you and how to enhance it and provides good inspiration to work towards your goals. Melting fat? All right, this is working. Gaining weight? Let's see what needs adjusting and implement it.

Getting conscious of where you are and at what point you are in your journey will create awareness and positive life changes. You can only fix something if you know what's wrong. If figuring out where you are and how you should start is challenging, consider consulting your professional health practitioner to assess exactly where you are now.

You could book an appointment to arrange blood work & urine samples to check your female hormonal health, heart, kidney, thyroid, digestive and nutritional health. Also, discuss the timing and dosage of medications you must take during such a fast. Finally, arrange your follow-up visit and how best to track your progress.

To measure yourself and promote self-discipline, you can make achieving your daily, weekly, or even monthly goals more inspiring and exciting by treating them like a game! For example, reward yourself after a job well done. You know you deserve it. Then, consider making it a group project, involve family members and friends of at least five people, and see who releases the most weight by the end of the week.

To keep track of the types of food you are eating, photograph your food before you put them into your mouth. It will make the difference between five chocolate bars and five carrot sticks. It will make you conscious of your food choices to implement the best options. Besides this, you could take at least five photos and measurements of your body. That way, you will keep tracking to reinforce that you are not just trying something out but purposefully reinforcing that this will work. It proves discipline in a game rigged for you to win. Through all this, be consistent with the measuring tools you use!

Ease Into Intermittent Fasting

Now that you know how to set the foundation, you can begin your intermittent fasting journey immediately. Note that fasting is something only some can do alone, especially if you are already unwell or suffering from specific mental and physical degeneration requiring additional assistance. Seek the help of a caring, qualified health physician for personal guidance on your intermittent fasting journey. Are you a growing child, pregnant or breastfeeding woman, under weight, starving, and deprived of proper nutrition? No! Any capable and healthy adult can incorporate intermittent fasting into their life and track how it works.

So, good news, you all are in all the way. Dance with me for 30 seconds.

Fasting is any period when you don't eat. Easing yourself into IF mode is no arduous task. Simply start with the following steps:

- Begin by cutting snacks from your diet for about three days. Stick to the basics, like breakfast, lunch, and dinner.
- Next, you can move on to a 16-hour fast or time-restricted eating schedule. During this period, you can have green and herbal teas and maybe even coffee with some cream. But be sure not to add any sweeteners. This fasting

method is very lax, but proceeding to a level-up is okay if you are ready for a challenge.
- You extend your fasting window by 30 minutes to an hour per day, consider drinking more water frequently, and reduce other beverages. Remember, a fast is voluntary, and you are always in control. While persistence is critical, if it's making you ill, eat your planned healthy meal.
- Continue to fast to make it a habit routinely. It is initially challenging, but the rest will come more naturally once you get the ball rolling.
- Water will become your best friend during these periods of intermittent fasting. Be sure always to keep yourself hydrated. Sipping on water will make your fasts easier to bear by outwitting your body with the illusion of fullness.
- Keep yourself busy to take your brain off the food! An empty mind is a devil's playground, and idle hands are a constant snacking hazard. You'll probably get a few funny looks from friends and colleagues who eat their square three meals a day at random times but be sure to stand your ground. You are an adult. You make your own decisions, which is a boundary you choose to keep. They will forget your peculiar patterns in a day or two.

Conquer Overeating

Proverbs 23:19 -21 says:

Listen, my son, be wise, and set your heart on the right path. Do not join those who drink too much wine or gorge themselves on meat, for drunkards and gluttons become poor, and drowsiness clothes them in rags.

While God put us on this earth to enjoy its various bounties, overindulging never did anyone any good. When people think of nutrition deficiencies and undernutrition, their minds often dart to images of kids in Africa with their stick-like arms and lack of food resources. Yet, I also think of the Hebrew captives in Auschwitz whose bones were cleaved to their skin like skeletons and sunken eyes when forced to sit at long outdoor tables with insufficient garbage meals slopped before them and the ashes raining down on their foods. Their appetites turned off, and their systems shut down, knowing that the ashes from the crematoriums and ovens were their relatives. But there is more to being nutritionally deficient than a lack of food resources.

This concept of 'The Overfeeding Paradox' exists, which dictates that while some people might be overfed, they are still undernourished. Studies show that obese people tend to face deficiencies in essential vitamins and minerals. The term' modern malnutrition' describes this trend, whereby overweight people suffer from the same nutritional inadequacies as those who are underweight and don't have consistent food sources.

Therefore, it becomes crucial to understand that your diet needs to consist not just of any food but of high-quality food. At all times, give priority to quality over quantity. But, again, even good things in excess can turn sour. If you go all out and eat excessive portions of healthy food within the times of your intermittent eating window, it still causes harm. Binging on healthy food is better than binging on unhealthy food, but it's like picking the lesser of the two evils. You could even develop a binge-eating disorder characterized by eating excessive food in one sitting. So be sure to eat healthy portions during your eating window.

If you find that binge eating has become your norm and feel like it's getting more out of your control, apply the following simple tips to contain your urges:

SELF-REFLECT

Binge eating can devolve into a disorder when you have not addressed the root cause of why you engage in it. Look deep within and ask yourself why you must eat so much at such times. What emotions and circumstances fuel this incessant craving to succumb to this activity? By being more reflective about your actions and intentions, you will better control the situation and your actions. Be your own master.

Do not starve yourself

Prioritize healthy meals containing vegetables, protein, healthy fats, and fiber-rich foods so you get a good dose of your daily nutrients but do not restrict your diet too much. If you suffer from a binge-eating disorder, seeking professional guidance to mitigate the issue is best.

Find a sound support system

A friend in need is a friend indeed. Surround yourself with a network of friends who support your recovery to regular eating habits. Suppose you hang out with people who constantly make you doubt your self-worth or are preoccupied with having ideal Instagram-perfect body standards. In that case, it is undoubtedly time to reconsider the company in your inner circle.

Work to manage your stress

Stress always leads to a mess. When you're stressed, you start craving snacks, which tends to be especially bad for binge eaters. Adopt the above-talked-about habits to destress yourself and eat fruit or protein when you have a stress snack attack urge.

Start eating intuitively

Eating distracted by a TV/laptop screen or even while working often leads to not realizing when to stop eating. Is it causing you heartburn and ulcers? Instead, eat upright at a table, slowly savoring and salivating your food, chew 47 times and taste each bite. Doing so increases your meal satisfaction, being more mindful of what is going into your mouth and controlling your food intake better.

. . .

TO GET STARTED with your intermittent fasting journey, start preparing in advance. Write down what your goals look like. Not everyone wants to lose weight. You might even want to fast intermittently to adopt a healthier lifestyle. Determine what part of your lifestyle needs fixing and pursue the ultimate results of your desirable aspects: sleep, stress management, relationships, eating habits, exercise regime, and spiritual fulfillment.

4

CONSCIOUS INTERMITTENT FASTING FORMULA: WHEN

Step 1

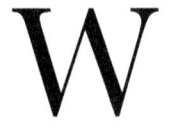

With the basics now covered, we can move on to the main course, or the lack thereof.

REASONS TO FAST

Firstly, we fast to overcome the emotional attachment to food. So, next time you pick up a candy bar or ice cream, ask yourself why? Could it be because of your childhood connection attaching the receipt of food to the love received from relatives, or are you emotionally hurt or excited, working hard and deserving a treat? Then, while you eat it, ask yourself how you feel and why you feel this way about this food and journal your answers. Exercising this muscle helps you understand why you choose certain foods and how to adapt to higher eating quality and be in control of food.

Secondly, the reason is to cleanse the body and rid it of heavy, fatty foods, eliminate excessive sweets, and prepare it for a selection of whole grains and vegetables high in fiber, which is beneficial to the colon.

Thirdly, purify the body before changing your diet to better your health. Intermittent fasting is the opportunity to teach your body what to eat.

Fourthly, to cure mental and physical stagnancy such as depression, fatigue, apathy, poor appetite, and unquenchable cravings for unhealthy foods and beverages requiring us to eat until we fall asleep. These persist into chronic ailments.

Fifthly, strengthening our spiritual prayer and meditation. Fasting draws you closer to God and frees you from burdens and addictions. People are reporting freedom from nicotine and alcohol with no physical withdrawal symptoms.

I am finally free from sugar, milk, ice cream, and cheese addictions. In addition, hope, courage, and new direction for any significant life goal such as career, finances, relationships, etc., replaced bad emotional habits, bondage, fear, depression, and negative insecurities. God opens doors that no man can shut. Fasting frees up cash and allows you to be generous to others. It beautifies you and restores your health. With all the disasters, predators and evil looming in the world, God extends His protection to you and your household when you pray and fast.

Sixthly, fasting enhances sleep, dreams, mental acuity, and awareness.

Fasting Methods

There are several intermittent fasting methods that you can implement.

Time-Restricted Eating

This fasting method requires you to introduce windows within which you will fast and eat throughout the day. So, if you were to fast for 12 hours a day, you are allowed to eat for 12 hours - 12/12 routine.

If you wish to undertake intermittent fasting for the first time, this method might be the thing for you. Some of this method's most common time variations are:

- The 14/10 routine: eating only in a window between 09:00 and 19:00 hrs.
- The 16/8 routine: eating only in a window between 10:00 and 18:00 hrs.
- The 20/4 routine: choose 4 hours in the day you will eat.

Whether you do it once or twice a week or decide to do it every day, if you are very active, it becomes essential to take most of your calories before the sun sets where viable. That is because we eat more low-nutrient, calorie-dense foods at night. So not eating at night allows our blood sugar to normalize before bedtime.

5:2 Method

As the name might suggest, two days per week, this method requires you to carefully look at the calories you are consuming and put a cap on it at 500 calories. During the other five days, you can freely eat healthy foods whenever you want. These two fasting days can comprise meals with 200-calorie and 300-calorie meals. Keeping them high in fat, fiber, and protein will allow you to fill your belly and keep your calorie count low. You can do this Monday, Wednesday, Friday, and Sunday, ensuring a non-fasting day between the two fasting days.

Alternate Day Fasting

This method requires you to fast every other day. You could also modify your manner of fasting in a way that is most comfortable for you. For instance, reduce your calorie intake to about 25% of your daily consumption. Then, on non-fasting days, resume your regular intake pattern, considering quality over quantity. Other stricter variations of this approach also call for consuming 0 calories on alternate days rather than the usually prescribed 500.

One Meal A Day or OMAD

Intentionally skipping a single meal is a cringe factor for most people dead set on eating 6 square meals daily. However, fast for 23 hours, including sleep time, is 23:1. It seems excessive, so why would you do it? Freedom from planning meals, and calorie logging, eliminates the sluggishness after eating lunch and makes you more productive and focused. You get to eat one meal, consisting of whatever you want, ensuring optimal fuel for the body. Most people choose to eat it around dinnertime. It builds your fasting and discipline muscle. It puts cells under stress and improves the body's resistance to disease. You can utilize this method every other day by incorporating it into Alternate Day Fasting to assist with any ravenous feeling and prevent binge eating. Doing so will also alleviate low energy, brain fog, fatigue, and physical weakness. Do not engage OMAD if you will eat two or three meals in a single meal. If you have firm discipline, eating between 11:00 – 13:00 hrs support the advanced development of mind and spirit and drives the liver and its subtle metabolic processes to work most efficiently.

This method also builds your fasting muscle to do extended water-only fasts, lowering the risk of cancer and diabetes. So why not incorporate it every other day or once per week?

24-Hour Fast or Eat-Stop-Eat Method

This fasting method is done once or twice a week and requires 24 hours of non-stop fasting. The most common methods include fasting from breakfast to breakfast or from lunch to lunch the following day. As one might expect, due to the rather extreme nature of this fast, people who jump right in tend to feel the burn and side effects like fatigue, headaches, irritability, and low energy. Drink water.

While all these recommended methods yield varying results, the Time Restricted Fasting method generates the best returns for beginners. It is the most sustainable and helps you develop more critical thinking regarding your food and schedule. You choose what you eat, when, and why you will eat. It might be tedious at first, but this fasting method helps you train both mind and body not to eat all the time and not eat unhealthy foods. In addition, research has shown how one fast determines the changes in metabolism throughout the day. Therefore, this time-restricted fasting can help you time your IF for maximum effectiveness.

The compelling reason why so many people opt for IF is that it meets you where you are. You can adjust it according to your convenience. For instance, if you've tried an IF window that makes you dizzy or hangry, eat earlier and adjust the window accordingly. Investigate to understand your body's Circadian Rhythm and tailor your fast for the most effective results from your fast. This fasting method aligns when and when not to eat with your body's internal clock and strongly emphasizes an earlier eating window.

It works in a way that narrows one's eating window to daytime hours and relegates the fasting to the night hours. While night and day would divide the fast into 12/12-hour sections, the fast part can also be extended into 16 hours, making the eating window 8 hours. A classic textbook circadian fasting method would have an eating window from 10:00 to 18:00 hrs followed by a 16-hour fast from 18:00 to 10:00 hrs the next day.

THE EARLY TIME **Restricted Fasting method** also caters to those who dread missing breakfasts, limiting your eating window between 08:00 to 14:00 hrs. With seven days to adjust, it yields even better results than regular time-restricted fasting, with more incredible benefits for insulin resistance, weight loss and other improved metabolic parameters.

. . .

WHILE QUITTING your IF halfway through may be increasingly tempting, especially if you think it is not working for you, don't hesitate to change it! There are various methods and techniques you can adopt to motivate yourself. For example, using clocks on paper, one such manner is to shade the fasting and feasting window. Doing so will visually reinforce the decision about designated fasting time distinctly from eating.

Rev-Up Metabolic Flexibility

ANYONE WHO PLANS to start losing weight must note that dieting indefinitely is not a long-term option. After the initial dramatic loss, the weight loss soon plateaus. This whole weight loss process must follow two steps that tackle the body's insulin levels. First off, the quality factor must be feasible. 'What' we eat is a considerable part of weight loss. Secondly, 'when' we eat is directly connected with the long-term problem of insulin resistance, a precursor of type-2 diabetes, metabolic inflexibility. When you eat carbohydrates abundantly, your cells do not open to receive the fuel. The symptoms are feeling hungry, extremely thirsty, frequent urination, frequent infections, fatigue and tingling hands and feet—reverse insulin resistance with intermittent fasting and a low-carb diet.

It is critical to understand the concept of metabolic flexibility. Metabolic flexibility is the ease by which the body switches between burning fat or carbohydrate as fuel derived from food or fuel already stored in the body to support health and wellness. The body's ability to seamlessly shift from one source to another improves fat-burning, controls blood sugar, and sustains energy. However, eating three meals a day plus snacks makes the body crave carbs for energy, inflexible and hungry.

After eating your last meal and fasting all night while sleeping, your metabolism switches to the fuel already in the body to activate the fuel-burning process of fat oxidation, which is burning fat. The body will metabolize the next meal you eat and use it for energy, where it burns sugar, termed glucose oxidation.

As soon as you eat a meal, the body automatically begins to store the first 1000 calories as fat in the liver and muscles as glycogen and simultaneously uses the rest for energy production. Then, during fasting, it switches to burning the fat or sugar fuel already stored. Depending on how you feed your body, you can be a sugar-burner which is a person who consumes a high-carb diet or a fat burner which is a person who consumes a whole foods diet, eating primarily non-starchy vegetables, high-quality proteins and healthy fats, limited fruits, and does not require food all day.

The transition period is 2 - 7 days to switch from sugar burner to fat burner. Metabolic flexibility is how IF works. It makes your body release energy from fat deposits and other energy sources while fasting.

While intermittently fasting, the first seven days are crucial as they will put your body into a self-induced state of ketosis. Your body will, during this time, begin to burn fats instead of glucose for energy. During this time, you will likely feel fewer snack cravings and more mental clarity, inspiring you to go further in your journey. Two of the most crucial things you must remember during this process are a strict ban on snacking and a lower-carb eating plan.

Once you have gotten into the fasting rhythm, you can optimize your fasting schedule and create your fasting and feeding window for the next 27 days. During this phase, you will customize your feeding window to capture healthy carbohydrates from green and starchy vegetables, legumes, whole grains, and fruits.

Whether you are in peri-menopause, menopause, and coming out of menopause, you will follow the formula to eat food sequentially that optimizes energy output, melt fat and longevity. However, women in peri-menopause still experiencing menstruation can select and time their macronutrients, fats, proteins, and carbohydrates, depending on the part of their cycle.

Intermittent Fasting During Peri-menopause

Allow me to explain.

Our monthly cycle consists of three stages: follicular, ovulatory, and luteal. Each month's cycle ends with menstruation, in which your uterus sheds its lining, making you bleed, typically for one to five days. So, your IF should be customized based on these three phases:

FOLLICULAR

This phase is when your body prepares for a fertilized egg. Estrogen levels are initially low but start increasing to prepare for ovulation. To support yourself during the follicular phase:

- Eat zinc-rich foods, like seafood.
- Eat foods containing phytoestrogen to maintain healthy estrogen levels, like cabbage, cauliflower, and garlic.
- Intake enough omega-3 fatty acids from sources like fatty fish
- Have lighter meals consisting of broccoli, green leafy vegetables, cauliflower, and more.

OVULATORY

The ovulatory phase kicks in when your body releases a mature egg for a potential pregnancy. This phase deals with increased levels of estrogen, testosterone, and progesterone. For support during this phase:

- Eat food rich in vitamins B and C.
- Consume fruits and vegetables rich in phytonutrients like spices and fresh herbs.
- Include cruciferous vegetables.

- Consume healthy fats like seeds, avocados, olive oil, and coconut oil.

Luteal

This phase covers the last 18 to 28 days of your monthly cycle. There is a decline in estrogen levels. For support during this phase:

- Include minerals like magnesium and selenium in your diet.
- Consume omega-3 fatty acids.
- Focus on B vitamins.

The first 21 days of the cycle are the best time to fast, assuming you have a regular 28-day cycle. Remember:

- Avoid fasting if you plan to get pregnant because, at this age, you still can.
- Consume plenty of nutrients during your feasting window.
- Guard your stress levels. Schedule 3 meals and skip snacks if you are under much stress.
- Hydrate yourself with magnesium, calcium, potassium, and sodium electrolyte minerals.
- Eat more protein, particularly grass-fed and organic.
- Consume healthy fats from olive oil, coconuts, seeds, and avocados.
- Avoid alcohol, processed sugars, caffeine, and spicy food.

Intermittent Fasting During All Phases

The next step to your fasting journey is to expand the fasting window and bring variations into your fast that would benefit you even more. At this stage in your fasting journey, your body will withstand a 24-

hour fast better. As a result, you can expect an increased fat loss, fewer night-time cravings, increased insulin sensitivity, reduced inflammation, improved mental clarity, and the list could go on.

Hydration Formula

While eating is restricted, planning what you will drink in your fasting window and how much water you will ingest is crucial. The short answer would be a lot. Drinking water during intermittent fasting is not only super important for general health and well-being, but it is also crucial for the success of your intermittent fasting. Water carries nutrients and oxygen to the body's cells, preventing constipation. In addition, since the menu requires you to eat high-fiber foods, fats, and protein, abundant hydration helps facilitate proper digestion and prevent digestive discomfort when starting your new schedule.

On the general recommendation to drink half your body weight in water in ounces daily, drink 60 ounces if you weigh 120 pounds. You could also drink 6-8 cups of water daily. Some professionals might even recommend drinking a milliliter of liquid for every calorie consumed. Listen to your body and stay hydrated throughout the day. That means drinking water when you are thirsty.

In addition to water, teas can aid your weight loss journey. Studies on green, black, Pu-erh and oolong tea have found that these teas may enhance weight loss and help fight belly fat. Brewing loose non-fruit herbal teas such as cinnamon, mint, ginger, and chamomile is aromatic. Your fasting liquids may also comprise water with salt and electrolytes. While excess coffee may be associated with adverse bodily side effects, plain coffee decreases appetite and increases metabolism. When drunk in moderation, it aids your weight loss journey.

While you may still lose weight, skipping all indulgent foods during your fasting window is best to achieve all the benefits of autophagy. These include vitamins, supplements, non-caloric flavored drinks, non-caloric sweeteners, sugar-free gum and mints, essential oil, lemon, lime, apple cider vinegar, milk, and cream. I also abstain from bone broth, soup, sugar, honey, coconut oil, MCT, butter, BCAA, energy drinks, and protein meal replacement shakes. Feel free to grab them during the eating window.

Besides these basics, studies have shown that drinking lemon or apple cider vinegar in warm water at night boosts your metabolic rate. They help the body burn fat, control hunger, balance glucose, and increase energy. These drinks also help regulate blood pressure, reduce bad cholesterol, help with digestion, and cleanse the liver and lymphatic system. I have a warm cup with each meal.

While the list of things you can drink may be extensive, the list of not-to-drink is even longer but relatively simple to follow. The basic rule is this. You must, in all cases, avoid adding sweeteners and creams to your drink as they beat the point of keeping food fast.

The Jet Lag Relief

If you travel a lot on airplanes and trains, and your generally lengthy transportation and transit time coincides with the fasting window, make changes just for that time. Make a conscious decision before traveling to either stick to the fast or vary the time and adjust the clock to feel your best. For example, forget the peanut bags or the quick sandwich on the plane. Snacking is a big no-no. Instead, scientists have recommended fasting for 16 hours before your plane touches down or your train reaches your destination. Fasting for 16 hours will help you reset your body clock and facilitate easy adjustment when arriving at your destination.

Celebratory Events

Life happens - birthday parties, weddings, Christmas, and Thanksgiving. Set your intermittent fasting schedule accordingly. It would help if you planned to vary the eating window by revisiting the clock and purposefully adjusting it to make it easy. If you choose to fast during some events, avoid stepping on any toes by being too fussy about it. Instead, focus on proper etiquette in communicating with people and building relationships. While not eating, engage in other activities that may make people feel comfortable around you. Take this opportunity to show off your attentive listening skills.

Medication And Supplements While Fasting

Consult your health professional before modifying, halting, or changing your medications. If you take prescription medication, intermittent fasting will affect your regimen. Intermittent fasting increases or decreases the effectiveness of your medicines by inhibiting or enhancing your body's absorption rates. In other words, fasting increases the side effects of certain drugs and supplements. Additionally, if you suffer from low blood pressure and are on medication, fasting without supervision is dangerous if not adequately addressed. Enlist the help of a medical professional before starting.

Issues to address are which method to begin with, the timing of the fasting and eating window, the medication dosage, and the timing to incorporate them. They will assist with associated issues and with eliminating medication eventually.

Supplements disrupt autophagy. Fasting is a welcomed stressor on the body to allow the cells that are scavenging for fuel to adapt to oxidative stress that elevates the longevity gene expressions SIRT1 and SIRT3. The antioxidants in multivitamins and water-soluble vitamins like vitamin C does the work instead of the cells. Fats like MCT oil and soft gels containing cod liver oil, fish oils, omega-3, and fat-soluble vitamins A, B_1, E, D, K_1 and K_2 break the fast. Branched Chain Amino Acids (BCAA) contain leucine which is insulinogenic because it triggers beta cells within the pancreas to release insulin. CoEnzyme Q10, Protein powder, and pre-workouts break the fast.

To optimize absorption, here are ways to take supplements. Water-soluble vitamins absorb better with food. Greens and fat soluble vitamins absorb better in fatty foods. However, to pull excess calcium out of the soft tissues into the bones, it is better to abstain from dairy so that there is no interruption while taking fat-soluble vitamins D3 and K$_2$. Stomach acids such as enzymes and apple cider vinegar pills can be taken before food, while it is best to take alkaline bile salts after a meal. Minerals need acids to absorb, so electrolytes are best taken on an empty stomach. Finally, take calcium and probiotics before bed.

Common Fasting Mistakes

I'm sure you're eager to begin your intermittent fasting journey now, having heard about its beautiful benefits. But, as excited as I am for you, there are certain things you must bear in mind to make your fasting effective and ensure you are investing your time and effort in the right direction.

Do not overeat **when you finish a fast regimen**

While it may be tempting, you will undo all that hard work for nought if you throw it away in a buffet right after following through on your regimen.

Eating too **little can also be a problem**

Fasting is a conscious choice over which you are in control. There are better ways to go about fasting than starving yourself. A controlled eating formula aids your body's well-being. The goal is not to take away nutrients. It's to enhance and narrow down nutrient intake to the most essential. Not eating is as bad as overeating.

Don't eat **unhealthy food during your eating window**

Your menu must contain healthy fats, carbohydrates, and proteins for optimal health. This menu builds your body and starves off infections, bacteria, viruses, and diseases. To do otherwise feeds them.

. . .

Dehydration and Deprivation

Do you ever feel willing, but your body drags during a workout? Not drinking enough water can imbalance energy levels and make you feel sluggish. Unfortunately, it can also lead to overeating, weight gain, slow metabolism, mental fog, and moodiness. The body consists of 60% water, which needs topping up daily to fuel cells that enable your body to function optimally and prevent headaches, constipation, urinary tract infection and kidney stones and prevent your fitness from plateauing. Unfortunately, you really can't get enough water.

Lifestyle choices must go in tandem

Fasting, bar hopping with friends the next night, and waking up at odd hours won't do any favors. Instead, regulate your lifestyle choices during this time of fasting and work to enhance your weight loss journey. Ladies have used IF to combat alcohol addiction altogether. What else can you achieve?

Giving up when results aren't immediate

Good things take time! If your fast isn't working, give it a few more weeks. If it is still not working, consider modifying them as depicted. Giving up would do no one good, especially you! You've got this!

Here is your first step to intermittent fasting. Start by choosing a suitable fasting method. In the case of peri-menopause, the first 21 days of the cycle are the best time to fast. Hydrate by drinking half of your body weight of water in ounces daily. Consider the recommendations for medicating and supplementing during intermittent fasting and avoid making common fasting mistakes.

5

CONSCIOUS FEASTING: WHAT TO EAT

Step 2

Food is fantastic. It identifies human culture. As modern people, cuisines and foods that might have been hard to procure are now readily available, especially if you live in a metropolitan city. Being spoilt for choice, you must refrain from indiscriminately gorging on anything you get your hands on. Your love for pork could be killing you!

Let's look at foods, what to add to your diet, and what to cut out. You will surely appreciate your body better with a better understanding of food. Soon, you will regain control over your body.

Intermittent fasting is easy when I reveal the simplest ways to start by luxuriating through the unrestrictive Mediterranean eating plan in a relaxed feast window. Most people prefer it because it works well long-term. Besides this is the push-it section in which the prescribed low-carb diet is very restrictive.

Once the fast part is over, here comes the question of how to break the fast. Yes, even breaking the fast is a process that requires time and patience. As much as you would like to jump into eating snacks and ordering takeout, it would help if you resisted the temptation not to undo your days/months of hard work.

So, how to break a fast? Experts have extensively researched the topic and believe that the foods you start eating, especially after a fast are vital. They could work to either amplify your fasting gains or sabotage and cause increases literally.

Breaking a Short Fast

18:6, 16:8, and 14:10 are some of the most famous and often used IF methods that require you to not eat within 18, 16, and 14-hour windows, respectively. While breaking this short-term IF pattern does not require as much forethought as extended fasts, you must remember some general rules of thumb.

Sticking to whole foods and going for a proper mix of macronutrients instead of reaching for a brick of carbs while on an empty stomach must be a priority numero uno. Prevent blood sugar roller coasters by avoiding sugary drinks and carb-loaded meals, raising your insulin levels, and making you hungrier.

Instead, you should break your fast with a low-glycemic meal or foods promoting low blood sugar. If you want to add carbs to your food, balance it with sufficient proteins and fats. When you do intense time-restricted eating plans like the 20:4 or the 18:6, portion size becomes essential. At all costs, avoid eating huge meals too fast, as they overload your digestive system and result in bloating.

Breaking an Extended Fast

As mentioned, the rules for breaking a fast become even more restrictive, especially if it is your first time ending an extended fast of 36 or 72 hours. Avoid excess sugar and carbs and eat easily digestible foods. Research shows that while you fast, your body stops producing the regular high volume of digestive juices needed for the digestive process. If you were to suddenly shock your body again and eat a lot in one go, it could result in inevitable discomfort and diarrhea.

Therefore, you must slowly but calmly ease your way back into eating food. Start with a nourishing soup and then move on to cooked veggies, which are easier to digest. Keep portion size in mind. Because that resulting lump in your throat, although it does not burn, is an ulcer.

Foods To Avoid After a Fast

While saying you must restrain yourself is all good, I will now provide you with a handy list of foods you must avoid at all costs and why.

Alcohol, processed sugary foods like candy, cookies, sodas, fruit juices, fried foods, foods with lots of salt, white bread and pasta, and processed meats like beef and deli meats work to increase your blood sugar levels and are generally very bad for your liver. These foods contain added sugars, saturated fats, and trans fats, which inflate inflammation.

On the other hand, add foods like garlic, turmeric root, leafy green vegetables, apples, green tea, beetroots & carrots, walnuts, lentils, avocados, tomatoes, and quinoa to your diet. Not only are they superb for lowering blood sugar levels, but their various properties are also exceptional for your liver.

Eradicate Bloating

You cannot take bloating lightly. It is the build-up of excessive gas in the intestines due to inadequate digestion of proteins, the body's inability to break down sugar and carbohydrates, and imbalances in gut bacteria. You can obliterate bloating in the following ways:

- Drink plenty of water throughout the day.
- Extend the fasting window.
- Finish the last meal 4 hours before bedtime.
- Consume probiotic supplements at bedtime.

- Eat some more fibre, including water-rich fruits and veggies.
- Prepare cruciferous foods with cloves of garlic to break down the hard-to-digest starches and sugars.
- Address the added sodium from dressings, condiments, carbonated drinks, savory snacks, cereals, and wines.
- Add natural diuretics to increase urine production to flush the extra sodium such as asparagus, green beans, pineapple, grapes, and watermelon.
- Limit empty carbohydrates.
- Avoid dairy products, sweet and sugary snacks, artificial sweeteners, chewing gum, and carbonated drinks.

Regeneration Formula After Cancer

As of today, cancer afflicts more than 25% of the American population. In addition, a disease that was once associated with old age now afflicts all age groups, including infants. Research traced such an increase in numbers to two main factors:

Environmental factors include:

- Increased sedentary lifestyle.
- Overeating of rich food.
- Depletion of the soil resources.
- Food processing.
- Omnipresent low-level radiation.
- Increased susceptibility to infections.
- Increased environmental toxins.

The second factor is the calculable statistical increase due to advanced diagnostic methods to identify cancer.

Research in the early twenty-first century has given rise to an ever-increasing consensus that certain types of chemicals, smoking tobacco, fried fatty foods, and insufficient vegetables and fruits in your diet all contribute to cancer.

Let me tell you about three increasingly popular rejuvenating dietary therapies that have been in the works for many years. They contain various combinations of foods that powerfully heal cancer and advocate whole foods and some animal products. However, only minimal amounts of whole fruits are allowed where required, and their juices must include fibre.

The first therapy consists primarily of grains, seaweed, microalgae, legumes, vegetables, herbs, sprouts, omega-3, gamma-linolenic acid (GLA) foods, oils, and minimal spices. Although raw vegetables or sprouts are desirable, most food on this list requires cooking. Therefore, fish and other animal products supplement it where necessary. The proportions are 40% unrefined complex grains; 30% vegetables; 15% fruit; 10% beans; 5% other recommended foods. This therapy will not only reduce levels of the toxic waste that feed the cancer cells, but it will also reduce the degenerative diseases in people who are weak, anemic, cold, and have other deficiencies.

The second therapy consists of whole fruits, vegetables and their juices, wheat-grass juice thrice daily, seaweeds, seeds, grains, omega-3/GLA foods, oils, and other appropriate microalgae, spices, and herbs that eliminate toxins and enhance immunity. The proportions are 30% sprouted grains and seeds, 50% vegetables and fruits and their juices, 10% cooked grain eaten once daily, and 10% other foods. This therapy eliminates the disease-producing toxins more quickly than the first and is most appropriate for people who show strength and intense pulses and have neither loose stools nor signs of coldness.

The third therapy is the same as the second, including the proportions, except that all the foods are raw except for the daily vegetable soup and all the grains are sprouted. This time, it requires cleansing, purgative herbs and frequent enemas. Supplementary proportions are daily juice dosage: up to 10 cups (80 ounces) of fruit and vegetable; wheat grass or barley grass thrice daily: 2 teaspoons powder (2 ounces liquid). This therapy rapidly reduces toxins and excess and is most appropriate for an often constipated, robust individual with a strong pulse who is extraverted.

These therapies are meant to be flexible allowing the patient to combine various parts to meet specific needs. Cancer is usually a complex mix of excesses and deficiencies, so the level of cleansing must be acceptable to the patient and their problems. Furthermore, supplementing 25 micrograms of vitamin B_{12} thrice daily with meals helps prevent cellular structure distortion due to cancer.

Additionally, people who suffer from long-term illnesses tend to develop several deficiencies. In such a case, emphasize foods that build on what is lacking: millet, barley, seaweeds, black beans, mung beans, and sprouts. The significant uses of various whole foods are therapeutic in treating cancer and its multiple symptoms and problems.

Evaluate Your Food Supply

While all the food you eat ends up in the same place eventually, some researchers have studied food efficacy one step further and now even look at how the foods that combine in your stomach work together. The fact is that certain foods pair well while others don't.

Research has shown that the standard American diet is close to consisting of two-thirds animal products, associated with the common misconception that vegetarian food has lower nutritional content. However, a diet composed of two-thirds plant-based products is close to a plant-based one.

Since I walk the talk and don't just talk the talk, I have seen that my life has become much healthier after switching to a plant-based diet. People who actively work to eat a balanced diet of whole grains, vegetables, fruits, quality fats and protein foods lose excess weight faster.

Additionally, research has shown that a plant based diet dramatically improves gut health and allows your body to absorb nutrients better. It supports your immune system and reduces inflammation. Fibers lower the body's cholesterol levels and work to stabilize blood sugar, making them great for good bowel management.

. . .

Unrefined Complex Whole Grains

We need to introspect and see why we eat the unhealthy way we do. But first, most of us need to eat more whole grains! Foods with whole grains are an excellent choice for a nutritious diet. They provide our diets with fibers, vitamins, minerals, and other nutrients that help balance and complete it.

The Dietary Guideline recommends that at least half of all the grains in your diet should be whole grains which provide vitamins that are very important for your overall health. Not only this, but they help with lowering high harmful cholesterol levels, lowering the body's insulin levels, lowering blood pressure, and creating a feeling of fullness that can significantly aid anyone working to lose those extra pounds and battling the midnight snackies.

Flaxseeds, barley, oats, and whole wheat also have naturally high levels of lignans. Lignans boost estrogen levels. While people already struggling with obesity should be alert, whole wheat assists women in easing menopausal difficulty.

Legumes

Packed with nutrients and low in calories, legumes and their fiber and protein content make you feel full faster! When your body uses carbohydrates present in legumes, it provides a steady stream of energy for your body, brain, and entire nervous system. Eating more legumes lowers blood sugar and blood pressure.

Legumes and beans also contain antioxidants that help fight against cell damage and prevent disease growth and rapid aging. In addition, it benefits the digestive system and helps prevent several deadly digestive cancers.

Vegetables and fruits

Diets with numerous vegetables and fruits are, surprise, surprise, perfect for you! Not only can it reduce blood pressure, but it can also reduce risk levels of heart attacks and strokes and prevent some types of cancer. Additionally, people who eat a veggie and fruit-filled diet have a lower risk of infections, digestive problems, good blood sugar levels, and healthy appetites. Berries rich in antioxidants, such as blueberries, strawberries, raspberries, and blackberries, do not raise blood sugar as much as other fruits.

Sea vegetables

Seaweed is the pre-eminent dietary source of iodine that supports your thyroid glands. Not only does seaweed contain iodine, but it also contains vitamins and minerals like vitamins A, B-complex, C, D, E, and K, calcium, copper, folate, iron, manganese, omega-3 fats, potassium, silicon, sodium, sulfur, and zinc. In addition, with anticancer properties that support blood sugar stabilization and cardiovascular health, sea vegetables provide antioxidant and anti-inflammatory support that protect your body from cell damage. Furthermore, they lower low-density lipids (LDL), the bad cholesterol in the blood, a marker for underlying health issues. Moreover, they delay hunger and help you to melt fat. Sea moss, a spiky sea vegetable, contains 92 of the 102 minerals in your body.

Mediterranean Style

The Mediterranean diet is a non-strict diet that emphasizes eating lots and lots of vegetables, fruits, whole grains, legumes, and olive oil, capturing all of the above. In it, fish is one of the primary protein sources. Fret not, though. Consuming eggs and poultry are allowed, while red meats are eaten infrequently as part of your main course.

The Mediterranean diet has many benefits. First and foremost, it has been repeatedly associated with lower LDL cholesterol, reducing the risk of heart diseases and strokes. In addition, its ample vegetable content contributes to strong bones, reduces the risk of Parkinson's and Alzheimer's diseases, and bestows those who follow it religiously with longer life. Other than all this, recent emerging research results show that this diet dramatically benefits people with depression, anxiety, type-2 diabetes, and some forms of cancer.

Planned Foods to Have Available Ahead of Intermittent Fasting

The best plan to adopt with regards to a Mediterranean diet would be to make one-quarter of your plate whole grains, half your plate filled with veggies, and serve the other one-quarter of your plate with the chef's choice of a quality protein, that is, the length, width and thickness of your palm. Be sure to add plenty of whole foods like fruits, vegetables, whole grains, nuts, legumes, fish, and olive oil. Also, make sure to swap out your red meats for fish most of the time. As you begin, you can add the fruits and vegetables you like and add new ones as your taste buds widen.

OILS

While we often associate fats with the negative, it is not a fat dirty word. On the contrary, it aids cell growth, protects our organs, and significantly influences our body's ability to absorb nutrients. Additionally, fats help contribute to the sense of fullness after a meal and prevent overeating. Oils like olive, flaxseed, coconut, avocado, walnut, sesame, and ghee are excellent oils with nutrients that could greatly supplement your diet.

Salt

While eating salts in excess is not suitable for you, incorporating salts like Himalayan salt and Celtic salt would be a win for your health. Salts other than those derived from the sea often come from underground salt deposits of the ancient dry seabed. They have no microplastics or pollution, which increases inflammation. They are suitable for your health because they are rich in minerals, promote overall nutrition absorption, are loaded with electrolytes, support digestive health, and have many other benefits. They produce hydrochloric acid in the stomach that kills off microbes, helps digest protein and assimilate minerals. In addition, salts help keep us hydrated. The adrenals and immune system need a certain amount of salt. If we are low on salt, the risk of insulin resistance goes up. Salt aids the sodium-potassium pump to power our muscles and nerves and give us energy. We need 1 to 2 teaspoons depending on activity level and how much we sweat.

Substitutes, Sugar and Sweeteners

If that sweet craving is not letting you be, you're lucky to be alive in the 21st century. There exist several substitutes you can have for sugar. Ingredients like honey, stevia, dates, applesauce and other fruit purees can substitute for sugar in your meal.

THE SECOND STEP in intermittent fasting is to determine what to eat. Add leafy vegetables, green tea, garlic, turmeric, avocados, tomato, and quinoa to your provisions. Avoid sugary foods like candy, cookies, sodas, and concentrated fruit juices. Stay away from alcohol too. To avoid bloating, drink enough water throughout the day. IF is the opportunity to teach your body what to consume. Take advantage.

Trim your waistline, fatten your wallet, and crush chronic disease with intermittent fasting—in only 27 days!

> *"I always believe that one woman's success can only help another woman's success."*
>
> — GLORIA VANDERBILT

You might recall that I mentioned in the introduction how dramatic the changes that peri-menopause and menopause bring can be.

Prior to menopause, keeping your weight within your ideal range was tough, but not *this* tough. However, when peri-menopause arrived, in addition to facing a spate of health changes, including IBS, headaches, and mood swings, those stubborn excess pounds began looking like they were impossible to get rid of.

Yet I managed to lose weight, feel fantastic, and save money while at it—thanks to intermittent fasting.

Few things fulfill me more than sharing life-changing tips and strategies with friends. Intermittent fasting was such a game-changer for me that I knew I wouldn't be satisfied by simply sharing it with my family and circle of friends. As such, I was motivated to write this book—to reach as many women struggling against weight gain, anxious eating, and the eternal cycle of yo-yo dieting.

Throughout this book, I have demonstrated how IF helps you melt your fat away and prevent a myriad of health issues—including Type-2 diabetes, heart disease, and brain death.

I have shown how it stimulates your body to create new cells, harmonizes your hormones, and resurrects the 12 systems of your body. I hope that other readers can not only achieve their weight loss goals but also grow in confidence and achieve optimal health and happiness.

If you have found this book to be a complete guide for everything other women need to embark on the road to better physical and mental health through fasting, then let them know how you feel.

By leaving a review of this book on Amazon, you'll help many more women stop seeing excess weight and illness as something they must passively accept.

Simply by telling them how this book helped you and what they can expect to find inside, you'll help them understand that they can take control of their health while also looking fantastic and making significant savings on their grocery bill.

6

DANCE TO THE RIGHT TUNE: ENOUGH IS ENOUGH

While we constantly receive directions on how many calories we should cut out, how many hours we must fast, and how often we must exercise, one thing that no one tells us is when to pull back!

Well, this is the time: now that we are rebuilding our bodies with real food and measuring our changes, we must head towards body composition.

To begin this journey, you must remember: that there is power in restraint! While each body is different, a universal law applies to all: Pareto Principle, a.k.a.; the 80/20 rule. This rule states that 80% of the changes or consequences are due to 20% of the efforts. It sounds diabolically opposite to what all those motivational videos tell you - "put in your 100% always!" However, if you think of a fruit-bearing plant, only 20% of the plant contributes to making 80% of the fruit!

Think of your body as the same. Minimized but conscious effort can bring about 80% of your significant changes. Such minimal but effective practices would be strength training. No, you don't need to slosh yourself with heavy weightlifting daily. Just three days a week is perfect. Compiling this with intermittent fasting can keep osteoporosis at bay and, in turn, strengthen your bones. If you find it too hard to use additional weights, you can also use your body weight, and you only need to do the minimum. "What do you mean?" I'm glad you asked. You do the minimum amount of training required but in consistent repetitions. Again, there is overwhelming evidence for outstanding results from performing just 5 minutes of daily exercise, including high-intensity interval training - HIIT. It is as simple as tracking what you do by counting the number of repetitions to achieve a desirable outcome. Can you complete 50 squats in less than 5 minutes? Yes, you can. Perform ten squats five times. How about 50 more after 30 seconds of rest? Now you have completed 100 squats in 3 m 42 s, tell me how you feel tomorrow.

Therefore, restraint is vital! Work smarter, not harder. Attune your body to the right rhythm, and losing weight and gaining fitness will no longer be unattainable.

Increasing Calcium Absorption: What, How and When

We had just gotten used to the idea of the minimum doing the most for us, and supplements right now might sound like a big add-on!

But, before you decide to skip this part, here is a fact for you: by the age of 35, most women, especially Caucasian women, are prone to develop osteoporosis: a degenerative disease of the bones that makes them increasingly weak, reduces strength and fitness, and lose bone tissue. So, how much bone tissue left by age 50?

In the short run, you might want to lose weight to look or feel better; however, you will compromise your health if you don't do it correctly. You develop bone diseases despite all these fasting, exercise, and strength training efforts. It might sound dismal, but this is to give you a glimpse of what most women suffer from without even recognizing it. I don't want to provide quick and shallow ways to transform your body in 7 days; instead, I want to give you insights into wholesome health, fitness, and a healthier way of living.

In most Western medicine, calcium is the most sought-after supplement recommended to women with bone fragility. And, if you think that bone fragility can never happen, I am sorry to break it to you. It can happen to anyone, irrespective of genetics or life history. However, the know-how of increasing calcium absorption into your body can help you prevent it and even reverse ill effects. Calcium-rich foods formed the backbone of East Asian medicine for centuries. You must have wondered how natives from East Asia have such a high life expectancy. Among other factors, actively incorporating calcium-rich foods in their diet is one of the reasons.

Interestingly, in East Asian healing traditions, calcium is derived directly from whole natural foods known for their cooling, relaxing, calming, and moistening attributes. It is the formula for relieving insomnia, thirst, nervous anxiety, and various overheated conditions. In Chinese physiology, the body fluids, blood, and tissues that calm the spirit, relax the liver, and moisten the lungs are undoubtedly infused with calcium and other minerals and corroborate with the Western practice of using calcium-rich foods that benefit the nerves and heart. While the primary benefit of calcium supplements is strengthening the bones in the Western diet, supplementing various whole foods and herbs that build structural aspects of the body and target to improve the kidney adrenal complex is the East Asian style.

It must be confusing to tear apart the historic utilities of calcium supplements for bone and kidney health. The only thing you need to understand is that there is one solution to all these unprecedented problems for your bone health and fitness: calcium metabolism. That is the movement and regulation of calcium ions in and out of the body via the gut and kidneys and between body compartments such as the bone, blood, intercellular and extracellular.

While calcium is abundant in all kinds of foods, dairy, fish, vegetables, fruits, grains and pulses, nuts and seeds, the body needs to metabolize the calcium. Eventually, women forced to take supplements to alleviate one symptom develop further complications. Usually, the total body calcium is good, but it's all in the wrong places because calcium supplements require hormones, chemicals, enzymes, and co-factors to push calcium into the bones.

Stop taking over-the-counter calcium supplements and consult your physician. It would be best if you only consumed them where there is an excellent reason. Numerous studies show that taking more than one gram of calcium supplement daily for stronger bones and general health increases cardiovascular risk by 20%. The Women's Health Initiative study showed that one gram of elemental calcium supplementation increases fatality between 15 and 22% with or without vitamin D supplementations. Renal failure patients take supplements daily, increasing their risk by 22%. Too much calcium is toxic. The calcium-alkali syndrome, where we consume too much calcium by drinking too much milk or antacids, has side effects not limited to poor appetite, psychosis, confusion, vertigo, kidney failure, and death.

Now that you know about calcium's utilities and are convinced, let's dig into how to incorporate calcium while improving its absorption. Three elements will guide you on this journey to gain the perfect calcium balance in your body.

You must have guessed the first one; vitamin D is a hormone essential for your bones irrespective of your calcium intake: true. However, vitamin D also effectively improves calcium utilization and absorption by 20 times and assists with melting fat!

Eating green plants, including microalgae, is a way of getting sunshine and vitamin D to the body. At the center of the chlorophyll molecule is magnesium. Chlorophyll enables calcium utilization. Other co-factors for calcium absorption, vitamins A, C, and phosphorus, are bioavailable in green plants.

The second one is vitamin K_2 (K_2). The body cannot undertake calcium metabolism without the presence of K_2. This fat-soluble vitamin needs fats to enable the body to absorb it. But most women are K_2 deficient due to lifestyle changes like engaging in low-fat diets, which came with malabsorption of fat-soluble vitamins A, B_1, D, E and K and consequently deficiencies when only a tiny amount of these is needed to be effective in the bloodstream.

Without vitamin K_2, soft tissues ossify because there is no method to move calcium. This deficiency causes calcification in the soft tissues and blood vessels and demineralization of bones resulting in osteopenia, fractures, osteoporosis, inflammation in the joints, which leads to degenerative joint diseases, tendonitis, bursitis, and arthritis, and insulin resistance, which leads to damage of the arteries, coronary artery disease, high blood pressure, diabetes, bad gums, and dental decay and more calcification where it is not supposed to be like plaquing in the stomach, kidneys, lungs, breast tissues, and cornea of the eyes rather than stronger bones.

The reason could be that there is a need for calcium to act as a band-aid to combat oxidation in that part of the body. For example, where women lack vitamin E, which attenuates oxidative lesions, and selenium and glutathione, the liver's primary antioxidants. This combination of low nutrients damages the tissues causing ischemia which is the lack of blood flow. So, calcium rushes to the rescue, deployed as a defense mechanism to coat the offender at the expense of clogging and plaquing the soft tissues or cocooning the threat in a pearl, effectively creating stones. In addition, calcium gathers in parts of the body that control pH, like the stomach and kidneys; for example, calcium deposits into the stomach when it becomes too alkaline due to insufficient hydrochloric acid. Then there are the smallest bacteria, called nano-bacteria, which hide in calcium shells for survival. They cause calcification diseases like periodontal disease, kidney stones, gallstones, and clogged arteries. Although antibiotics can be ineffective on these, fulvic acid may assist.

There are ten types of vitamin K, but the most important is K_1, known as phylloquinone, which comes from chloroplast in green leafy plant foods such as turnip greens, collard green, kale, spinach, cabbages, and microalgae. And vitamin K_2 known as menaquinone, come from two sources. That is animal sources and fermented products. It is also produced in the human gut in small quantities by turning K_1 into K_2. The K_2 sub-groups range from MK-4 to MK-13, depending on the length of their side chain. Of these, bacteria do not produce MK-4. Instead, bacteria produce MK-5 to MK-15, which have longer chains.

Seventeen vitamin K-dependent proteins transport calcium from the soft tissues into the bones and teeth. Vitamin K_1 is involved in coagulation and preventing bleeding. K_2 builds up the mitochondria to provide endurance and a lot of energy during exercise and is helpful in the prevention and treatment of neurogenerative diseases such as Parkinson's and Alzheimer's. While K_1 leaves the liver within 8 hours, it stores K_2 for up to 72 hours. K_2 plays a specific role in the blood vessels and bones.

K_2 activates the Matrix GLA protein (MGP), an inhibitor protein in the blood vessels. MGP stops calcium from forming in soft tissues by binding to calcium, pulling calcium out of the tissues into the bloodstream transporting them to the bones. MGP is produced in the smooth small muscle cells in the blood vessels, allowing vasodilation and vasoconstriction.

Two types of cells in the bones are the osteoblast and osteoclast. The osteoblasts mineralize and build strong bones by taking calcium from the bloodstream and pushing it into the bones. The osteoclast demineralizes and destroys the bones by taking calcium out. Vitamins D and K_2 activate the hormone osteocalcin to bind calcium to the bone and are also known as a bone-forming protein. In addition, K_2 encourages the bones to pull calcium from the blood vessels and transform them into bone tissue.

Vitamin K_2 tackles the root cause, such as insulin resistance. It prevents the arteries and joints from turning into bones. It regresses pre-formed calcification by rerouting calcium from going to the wrong places and pushing it into the right areas. It increases vascular elasticity, prevents heart disease, and builds and maintains healthy, strong bones and teeth. Our blood wouldn't clot in its absence, making wounds hard to heal, and bones wouldn't develop properly. It reduces the intensity of night sweats and disturbed sleep in menopause; even diabetic patients benefit from K_2 supplementation.

Culprits that deplete vitamin K_2 are antibiotics, low-fat diets, statins, mineral oil, gastrointestinal tract issues, liver damage such as fatty liver, inefficient amounts of vitamin K_1 to convert to K_2, or not consuming enough vitamin K_2. Low vitamin E levels combined with high sugar and high carb diet create oxidation, making harmful bacteria thrive. Low vitamin levels will also cause the body to ration all the vitamins available for actions actively involved in short-term survival only. For example, the body will allocate vitamin K to coagulation to stop any broken vessels and internal bleeding before it allocates any vitamin to remove calcium from the soft tissues. Blood thinners antagonize both vitamins K_1 and K_2. Long-term use calcifies the arteries, aorta, valve, and coronary artery and causes vitamin K_1 and K_2 deficiencies.

Derived from organ meat, egg yolks, chicken, cheeses, and butter, of animals that eat green chloroplast from natural grass. The grain-fed animal product would lack vitamin K_2 because grains do not have vitamin K_2. Vitamin K_2 must come from the original natural product provided by nature first for high levels to be present in the animal cycle. Fermentation products make vitamin K_2. For example, natto, a traditional Japanese fermented soybean food, is exceptionally concentrated.

Currently, mainly research labs conduct vitamin K_2 measurements. They look at the non-carboxylate proteins to identify whether there is a K_2 deficiency. The Rotterdam Study conducted on thousands of males and females over 55 looked at their outcomes from consuming vitamin K_2 over eight years. It found that the amount of K_2 and calcification had a direct correlation. More vitamin K_2 intake meant less calcification. Some studies show that consuming 32 micrograms reduces coronary artery disease, aortic calcification, and cardiovascular death by 50% and all-cause mortality, including some cancers, by 25%.

To utilize vitamin K_2, engage in healthy intermittent fasting with significant quantities of green vegetables, fermented products, quality fats, and grass-fed animal products. And consult your doctor to ascertain the dosage of vitamin K supplements required for your circumstance.

NHS recommends taking one microgram (mcg) a day of vitamin K for each kilogram of body weight. For example, a lady who weighs 60 kg intakes 60 mcg daily. Introduce two K_2 foods to your daily diet. Nutritious cod liver oil is rich in fat-soluble vitamins D and A. It supports bone health, improves eye health, reduces inflammation, reduces joint pain, and improves rheumatoid arthritis symptoms.

One tablespoon (5 ml) contains 41 calories, vitamin D: 75% of the RDI, vitamin A: 195% of the RDI, omega-3 fatty acids: 890 mg, fat: 4.5 grams, monounsaturated fat: 2.1 grams, saturated fat: 1 gram, and polyunsaturated fat: 1 gram. Now marketed with added vitamin K, the recommended vitamin D to K ratio is vitamin D3 10,000 IU with K_2 100 mcg of MK7.

Foods high in vitamin K_2:

- Fermented foods, especially natto, have MK-4, 5, 6, 7, and 8.
- Sauerkraut, buttermilk, hard and soft cheese, have MK-4, 5, 6, 7, 8, and 9.
- Animal liver, which includes goose pate, has MK-4.
- Grass-fed butter and grass-fed meat - chicken, beef, duck, egg yolks, and egg white have MK-4.
- Eel, mackerel, and salmon have MK-4.

The third one, magnesium, is closely related to vitamin D absorption in the body, which is a known fact. However, according to a recent study, abundantly supplied calcium and vitamin D while holding back magnesium caused one individual to develop a calcium deficiency. However, on reintroducing magnesium, the calcium levels increased sufficiently.

Arthritis is excess calcium stuffing the soft tissue while it is simultaneously lacking in the bones. Calcium tends to deposit excessively into the soft tissue rather than enter the skeleton, actualized in degenerative diseases of the skeletal system, heart, arteries, vascular system, kidneys, and brain, as in Alzheimer's disease. Calcium causes the muscles to contract. Magnesium relaxes the muscles. That is why magnesium supplements and magnesium-rich foods are necessary remedies to stop and prevent headaches, heart disorders, and menopause symptoms.

Required for over 350 metabolic reactions, the absence of magnesium affects many systems as it is essential for blood pressure regulation, energy production, muscle contraction, and nerve signal transmissions. Consider a deficiency if you have three or more of these symptoms: acid reflux, polycystic ovary syndrome, constipation and other digestive problems, thyroid disorder, mood disorders, migraine, cluster headaches, tension, type-2 diabetes, heart disease, arrhythmia, high blood pressure, sleep disorders, wired brain, inability to cope with stress, fatigue, anxiety, irritability, weak joints and bones, weak muscles, cramps, spasm, fasciculations, eclampsia, vasospasm, auras, dizziness, vertigo and craving for ice cream and chocolate. Chocolate contains a caffein-like substance called theobromine, is rich in oxalic acid, and inhibits the healthful mineralization of the body. Limit this habit by getting your magnesium levels up.

The benefit of eating supplements and magnesium-rich unrefined plant food, plus significantly reducing salt intake, is that it relieves all these symptoms, including all the side effects of menopause. Give it 30 days. The different types of supplements specialize in various ailments.

Type	Specialty
Magnesium Chloride	Relieves heartburn by producing gastric juices such as hydrochloric acid in the stomach, which declines with age, treats constipation and elevates low magnesium levels.
Magnesium Glycinate	A muscle relaxant that calms the body and promotes sleep. Rids insomnia and anxiety and regulates circadian rhythm.
Magnesium L-threonate	Gets past the blood-brain barrier for cognitive function, relieves depression and elderly brain diseases, and improves memory and ADHD.
Magnesium Malate	Rids chronic pain like fibromyalgia and chronic fatigue.
Magnesium Orotate	Supports the cardiovascular system by improving energy production in the heart and blood vessels.
Magnesium Taurate	Improves blood sugar and blood pressure, energy production and recovery of the nervous system at the muscular-skeletal level for athletes. This form relieves stress and detox waste from the muscles and prevents arrhythmia.

No wonder a cure for osteoporosis, arthritis and calcium deficiencies is a magnesium-rich diet of whole foods. Food sources include cacao which is undamaged by heat and untainted by sugar. Other food sources are dried seaweeds, rich in the complete spectrum of minerals, e.g., wakame, kombu, kelp, hijiki, arame; most beans such as mung, aduki, black and lima beans; whole grains such as buckwheat, millet, wheat berries, corn, barley, rye, quinoa, and brown rice bran; nuts such as almonds, and walnuts; seeds such as pumpkin, filbert and sesame seed; high chlorophyll foods, such as wheat and barley grass; microalgae such as spirulina, chlorella and wild blue-green Alphanizomenon; greens such as spinach; and fruits such as bananas, avocados, and dried fruits including figs.

Okay, enough with the facts. Let's get started with an action plan to increase vitamin D, K_2, and magnesium levels and improve absorption:

- Consume whole-natural foods and greens because they are rich in calcium, magnesium and vitamins D and K_2.
- Consume vitamins D and K_2 in the presence of healthy fats.
- Avoid abnormally high dosages of zinc supplements example, 142mg.
- Take vitamin D3 and K_2 with magnesium supplements and treat vitamin D deficiency during the eating window.
- Eat some raw vegetables like coleslaw and limit denatured, processed foods because they deplete magnesium levels.
- Carbonated drinks, including soda and seltzer water, deplete magnesium levels.
- Quit smoking.

Here are some easy recipes to increase calcium absorption-

1. The green and grain soup: This recipe dates back a hundred years and is of European origin. There are only

two primary ingredients: barley sprouts and kale. It would be best to have sprouts because sprouting increases the levels of vitamins A and C, the calcium co-factors in the seeds. Bring the soaked barley to a rapid boil, then simmer for 10 minutes and add the kale towards the end of the cooking process. Caution: if you are using whole barley, soak it for at least eight hours before preparing this. You can easily include this soup in your diet, which works wonders for chronic bone issues.

2. A soup of beans: Beans benefit kidney function in Chinese traditions, and the kidneys rule the bones! If you believe in ancient traditions, have a go at this bean soup. Use any soaked beans and add seaweed to the soup. Simmer on low heat and enjoy the wholesome goodness.

3. Bone marrow soup: Yes, bones strengthen your bones. This recipe is embedded in a Chinese belief, saying "like heals like." For this soup, you can use bones from any organically grown grass-fed animal, break them into smaller pieces and let them simmer for a long time to extract the marrow and the minerals. You can add acidic vegetables to this soup to enhance the taste.

4. Fish soup: No, this is unlike any other fish soup you have ever had. This remarkable fish soup uses whole fish like sardines and anchovies. The source of nutrients is the bones of the fish. Once fully cooked, the bones are soft and easy to chew. Use seasonings of your choice. This soup is handy for severe calcium deficiencies since the fish bone induces calcium renewal.

The importance of wholesome home-cooked recipes is monumental, especially compared to synthetic supplements. Starting at 35, women start losing bone tissue three times faster than men. As a result, calcium absorption gets weaker due to increased hormonal imbalances. Most women now take the widely prescribed estrogen therapy to counteract it. However, the source of such estrogen is mostly animals in forms such as Premarin. In addition, a side effect of such therapy is the early onset of breast, ovarian, and uterus cancer. Therefore, even though estrogen therapy can slowly increase calcium absorption, it's best to avoid it.

Not much of a chef in the kitchen? And all the above recipes sound too much to deal with? Fret not. I've gotcha. We will explore how you can naturally increase calcium absorption without chopping and cooking!

Recommendations for Increasing Calcium Absorption

Prevent loss before building it up

One smart way is to retain the calcium in your body and improve the build-up, but most people don't imagine it this way. The trick is to halt the calcium loss from your body in the first place. Walk daily, take breaks between work to stand up and move, and bear the weight of your body to resist further loss of calcium from your bones. Additionally, jump, land on your heels, and wait for 30 seconds, then repeat. Yes, adopt this original method before moving on to processes of increasing absorption.

Sunlight is your best friend

Vitamin D and calcium absorption by the body are interrelated. You can enhance one by increasing your exposure to the other. For example, exposure to some sunshine for at least 15 minutes daily triggers melanin and up-regulates calcium absorption in your body. What about winters with freezing temperatures when you are covered head to toe in fluffy jackets? During these seasons, make a habit of exposing your hands and face to the sunshine. Once you make your daily dose of sun habitual, there is no going back. You are bound to feel changes in your body, including your mood and motivation! To keep yourself on track, you can set a daily reminder to step out to soak in some vitamin D.

. . .

Natural calcium nutrition with no special additives

Just increase the number of grains, legumes, seaweed, and leafy greens in your diet. Make sure to fill at least one-fourth of your plate with these for each meal. In the long run, this has the best impact on your health.

Herbal supplements

At some point, we can all use formulated supplements, whether we appreciate or dislike them. Your physician may have already recommended it when you do not have enough calcium. Consult a physician for the appropriate dosage and advice on any medication interference. You can opt for alfalfa, kelp, dang gui, or horsetail capsules that help assimilate calcium. The high silica content of horsetail has a bone remodeling effect. Silica is already present in bones, and it improves the absorption of calcium. By enhancing collagen synthesis, silica improves bone strength and tissue cartilage formation, density, and consistency. Healthy collagen levels protect the kidneys and other organs and contribute to a healthy cardiovascular system, skin elasticity, and joints. Especially if you need to incorporate calcium-rich foods in your daily meals, these can be alternatives! However, patience is critical. You would need to wait a few months before seeing or feeling any noticeable changes in your body. Or endure the external side effects of gorgeous skin, hair, and nails. Again, inform your physician of your herbal supplements for specific guidance, including when to stop dosing and resume.

Slay low-fat products

I know it is a trend now to chuck wholesome whole-fat milk down the drain and replace it with skim milk. Well, don't fall for it. Skim milk is devoid of enzymes that impact your body's calcium absorption. So, it's time to return to grass-fed whole-fat cow and, if lactose intolerant, goat's milk!

. . .

CULTIVATE with fermented foods

Include natto, yogurt, kefir, and buttermilk to get your daily dose of vitamin K$_2$ to boost calcium absorption!

Exercise is Fictitious

Let me burst the myth for you. Exercise is a scam. It sounds so good when I say that. Who wants to hit the gym? But I did. I did all I could to pound out those stubborn pounds, but things were not adding up.

Hippocrates, the early Greek physician and the father of medical science, advised that we would find the safest way to health if we could administer each individual the adequate quantity of nourishment and physical training, not too little and not too much.

A recent study revealed that Americans are still plagued with the problem of obesity, although they exercise more than the global average. On the other hand, Italians and the Dutch, with their low exercise rates, are less obese than Americans. So, what exactly is going on?

The solution is different from exercise but calculating your total energy expenditure. Running on a treadmill for 45 minutes a day opposed to living a flamboyant sedentary lifestyle for the rest of 23 hours and 15 minutes of a day, will not take you anywhere other than a weighing machine with a continually deflecting pointer towards the right.

Total energy expenditure is the sum of a range of factors:

Total energy expenditure = basal metabolic rate + thermogenic effect of food + non-exercise activity thermogenesis + excess post-exercise oxygen consumption + exercise.

Here, the basal metabolic rate is a sum of a range of tasks like metabolic housekeeping tasks, including maintaining the vital organs, maintaining body temperature, keeping the heart pumping, breathing, maintaining brain, liver, and kidney function, and more.

I want to highlight that total energy expenditure is different from exercise. For example, the basal metabolic rate for a lightly active average female is roughly 3000 calories per day. So, even if you walk moderately, at 3 miles per hour for 45 minutes daily, you will only burn 104 calories, not even 5% of the total energy expenditure.

Traditional diet and exercise computed as fifty-fifty partners are far from the truth. Diet does 95% of the work, but exercise gets 95% of the attention; hence, weight loss has always remained unachievable. A study on 39,876 women, called the Women's Health Study, easily one of the most expensive and comprehensive diet studies, divided women into three groups. These three groups represented low, medium, and high levels of weekly exercise. After ten years, the study concluded that the group with intense exercisers lost no extra weight. Do we even need more concrete evidence than this?

However, did you know we lose fats and muscles equally during weight loss? You don't want to lose critical muscle mass like heart muscles. Therefore, 5 minutes of targeted exercise is vital to maintain muscle mass, protecting the heart and other muscles from deterioration. Yes, lying on a couch and watching that daily sitcom while stuffing your stomach with popcorn often feels like heaven, but ladies, we also need to get moving. Squat!

Now that we have established our case favoring nourishment and food let's see how whole foods can help you achieve the needed results.

7-day Challenge

Intermittent fasting melts fat even if you eat a large chunk of cake at every dinner. However, it is your privilege to fast forward to this PUSH-IT formula and engage for seven days to achieve unequivocal metabolic flexibility.

Firstly, the basics to lose 1-2 pounds weekly is to eat within your caloric range as follows:

If you weigh 200 pounds or lighter, calculate your current weight x 10 x 1.2 – 500 = your daily calorie consumption.

If you weigh 225 pounds and over, calculate your current weight x 10 x 1.2 – 1000 = your daily calorie consumption.

. . .

SET the standard for the missions you will achieve by implementing the easiest options from these guidelines to start your challenge.

GET MEASURED USING a consistent tool to remeasure

The weighing scale is the trickiest instrument you will ever use to measure your progress. Yes, I know, sometimes it gets to you and tests your sanity. "How did my weight increase by 2 lbs in 12 hours? I didn't even eat any heavy meals today. It doesn't make sense. My clothes even fit looser." But, when we see the number on the scale, we believe it without second thoughts. That's where the negative cycle begins. You measure your weight too frequently, and that too on a scale. Some days, it triggers your anxiety and releases cortisol, the stress hormone, making it more challenging to lose fat.

Listen to me. It's time to upgrade from your scale for the moment. I did the same, and then things changed. First, you need to track the correct numbers to see your progress.

You can do the skinfold test using calipers to pinch and measure the thickness of your body in specific areas. Alternatively, you can pull out the measuring tape and measure your neck, shoulders, chest, arms, mid-section, waist, hips, thighs, inner knee, calves, and ankles.

I recommend my personally tried and tested instruments - the DEXA, that is, Dual-energy X ray absorptiometry, a type of X-ray passed through the body. It costs around $50-100 per session. I went in for a bone density scan and walked out with intriguing information.

Here is your reason for doing it. Although osteoporosis can affect any age group, women over 50 are particularly at risk because as estrogen levels decline with menopause, bone density decreases too. Broken bones cause osteoporosis, but the denser and more robust the bones, the less likely they are to fracture. Some radiation travels through the body, while the tissues and bones absorb some. But bone density scans use low-level radiation that allows the radiographer to remain in the room. The computer collects the amount of radiation passed through the bones and compares this measurement to the bone density of a young, healthy female of your ethnicity. At the same time, you get to collect accurate information on your body composition, such as the storage of the muscle and fat mass in your body. The scan even distinguishes subcutaneous from visceral fat.

The next, more affordable option is the Air Displacement Plethysmography, also known as the BodPod, costing circa $40–50 and is an egg-shaped air-controlled chamber. Body density is body mass divided by body volume. Your age, weight, height, and gender are first programmed to measure your volume in this confined space.

Hydrostatic weighing, costing around $35-50, works with the Archimedes principle, which states that if you put an object in a tank of water, the object will displace water equal to its volume. The temperature of the water makes it easier or difficult for the person to float. Information gathered beforehand is the density of the water, the tare weight, and your weight. Fat and air make a person float, so you must blow all the air out underwater. Although muscle does not weigh more than fat, a person with more muscles will sink faster underwater because muscle is denser than fat. Hydrostatic weighing is the gold standard for underwater weighing.

Other methods like BodyMetrix assess your body mass index, basal metabolic rate, disease risk, and lean body mass and detect actual fat thickness through ultrasound waves technology.

In summary, if you open yourself up to the idea of alternatives and find the strength to surpass your weighing scale, you will be instantly much more precise about your actual progress and, in turn, will better direct your weight loss journey.

TAKE photos of your body

It might sound silly initially, but this is the most effective and satisfying way of documenting your progress over time. It forces you to face yourself in the mirror, accept your reality and creates an impulse to improve your situation. Humans are visual beings. Nothing hits us more than an image, whether the portrayal of the body we want or our current body.

Though initially uncomfortable, taking photos can become a great way to stay motivated. Sure, the first photo of your baseline will be challenging to look at and accept. However, the visuals could be so unacceptable that they push you to change immediately. There are specific real-life stories where people on the same journey as you were able to curb their impulsive eating by just looking at their current body photos. The photographs reminded them of their progress but also acted as an awareness that stress, eating that sugar-loaded slab right now, would jinx their progress so far and set them backwards. This awareness is sometimes more potent than a day of diet or exercise. Awareness of your real-time situation is your first and foremost step in this journey if you know you are halfway there.

I say this confidently because our psychology, most of the time, drives our actions. So as long as you have control of your mind, the rest becomes easy!

SET the clock for fast and feast

Harmony, Harmony, Harmony! That should be your motto in this journey. But unfortunately, most of us believe that we must diet every day and never break the cycle to succeed. Well, I will tell you a secret: you can cheat!

As long as your cheating is in a controlled zone, you can cheat. Pick a day in your week. I recommend Saturdays for eating all you want. Eating all you were craving is a great trick to help ease your mind and cravings and, most importantly, keep the cravings at bay during the week. Believe it or not, it lets you stay on track and regulate things. So eat that junk, munch on those calories, and enjoy the dopamine rush on Saturdays so much that you don't need to consume more waste for at least five more days. You can take Sunday to detox your body and reset it before you start your journey on Monday again! However, the catch is that you must write down what you are feeling before you eat each particular food while you are eating it and any memories of why you initially liked this food. Tracking the emotions and psychological reasons behind it will bring some perspective, and you may even give up this food for life. Trashing junk is ultimately the reason you are allowed to cheat. Track this in your journal and see where it takes you.

No white foods for seven days

Someone must have suggested this to you before me. You should have taken it more seriously. But, if you are willing to see how changes in diet affect your body, explore this small experiment. Cut off the following foods - all bread, all rice, yes, brown as well, cereals, pasta, potatoes, fried food with and without breading, and tortillas. Essentially anything white or white-derived. You will sense a change in your body after this week, and it might be that you won't go back to eating whites again, which happened to me! A medical reason whites aren't good for you is the industrial bleaching these foods go through. Through the bleaching process, the residual protein in these foods turns into alloxan, an inducer of diabetes! That's one reason enough.

Choose the recipes you will use for seven days and gather the ingredients not already available in the pantry

Another intelligent way of regulating your diet is this. Plan well and stick to the plan. Walk with me, step by step. First, plan out your calories and determine your nutritional requirements. Now you move on to planning your plates, i.e., meals. Each meal plan includes the ingredients you want on a plate and their calorie and nutritional profile. Finally, you shop for only the ingredients in the meals you eat throughout the week.

Now, it's important to remember the timing of your meal, the frequency, and the portion size. More than what you eat, you must have a minimum of 4 hours gap between two meals. So, there you go:

- Pay attention to nutrient profiles.
- Prepare your macronutrients of quality fats, carbohydrates, and proteins.

- Plan your meals the night before.
- Manage the timing between meals.
- Have balanced meals with the proper portion size.

And voila! You will start melting fat within the month!

Eat the same meals over and over

How does it feel when I tell you that you must repeatedly eat the same meals? I am sure you feel trapped. But consider this, how different are your meals every day? With hindsight, I won't exaggerate when I say that I repeat one to three meals every week, and I love it.

When I settle down, I eat a colorful three-course meal like in a restaurant. For example, I have starter protein soup, a main meal of assorted veggies and fish then my dessert followed by a lettuce salad or celery sticks. So, my meals are spiced to be nice. I sip on a warm cup of apple cider vinegar at each meal. It is during my mealtime that I consume my supplements. I enjoy one meal daily most days while I indulge in a four-hour eating window sometimes. When I see the progress I make this way, that keeps my stomach satiated for another week.

I had only one cheat day last month and am already melting the fat.

I suggest you mix and match from this initial list:

Proteins include free-range egg whites, grass-fed beef, chicken breast or thigh, and wild caught, fatty fish. Legumes consist of lentils, black beans, pinto beans, red beans, and mung beans. Vegetables include spinach, broccoli, cauliflower, peas, green beans, bok choy and more.

Some produce is heavily sprayed and tested high for pesticides even after peeling, washing and cleaning them. It is best to buy some organic produce to keep the chemicals out of your body, especially if you eat the skin while others protect themselves.

This list consists of foods that are best bought organic:
1. Apples, 2. celery, 3. cherries, 4. grapes, 5. kale, 6. nectarines, 7. peaches, 8. pears, 9. potatoes, 10. spinach, 11. strawberries, 12, sweet bell peppers, 13. tomatoes and 14. sweet corn.

This list contains products that you do not need to buy as organic produce:
1. Asparagus, 2. avocados, 3. broccoli, 4. cabbages, 5. cantaloupes, 6. cauliflower, 7. eggplants, 8. frozen sweet peas, 9. honeydew melons, 10. kiwis, 11. mushrooms, 12. onions, 13. papayas, 14. pineapples.

Hydrate each day

Drink water, water, water. Drinking enough water ensures that your liver works optimally to support fat loss. While "I don't particularly appreciate drinking much water" is a standard narrative among women, you must overcome such dogmas. Now that I look back, even I plateaued in fat loss, mainly because water intake was the last on my to-do list. As soon as I observed this error in my ways, I thought this could be the roadblock preventing me from losing weight. Hence, I added a few more glasses to my daily intake. As a result, my fat loss journey resumed, and I lost two pounds in the same week.

Here are my two cents: Ensure you drink even more water on your cheat day. Why, do you ask? The carbohydrate overload on your cheat day will require more water to function your digestive system properly. The lack of the necessary amount of water translates into headaches and constipation. No other beverage can facilitate healing like water.

Cut out sugar and sugar substitutes for seven days

Just chuck them in with the whites. Drink some magnesium if you are craving chocolate, and the thought of white chocolate sends creamy signals to your white fountain brain. You are guaranteed metabolic flexibility.

Cut out all dairy for seven days

I know it is challenging. Cutting down dairy for seven days is tough, especially if it is your addiction, as it was mine. You will find it more brutal when you finally realize the different forms of mucus-forming dairy that creep into your daily life, knowingly and unknowingly. But I will be completely unemotional here: cut that junk out.

Cow milk has a low glycemic index and a low glycemic load. But milk has high insulinemic indexes of 90-98. This jargon quantifies the typical insulin response to various foods. Remember I asked you to cut down on white bread. So, if you consume dairy, you consume a similar food with the same insulinemic index. Are you screaming for ice cream? Take magnesium.

Remove dairy; you will noticeably accelerate your fat loss journey. However, I know it is hard to survive without coffee. Quick solution, use cream instead of milk. But ensure not more than two tablespoons and remember it interferes with autophagy.

No fruits for seven days

Are you not allowed fruit too? You don't need to have fruits year-round. Tomatoes and avocados are permitted. But the idea is to cut down on fructose, its sugar content. Why? Habitual fructose consumption contributes to chronic diseases such as insulin resistance, diabetes, liver disorders, and obesity. The goal is to melt fat, so no fruits and no fruit juices, no, not at all.

No complaining: if you messed up, reset!

Have you messed up? It happens. Are we even following rules if we don't break them at first? But believe me. You will slowly get used to them and instead enjoy them. So, if you messed up a particular day or just gave up for any reason whatsoever, don't lose hope. Instead, reset and start fresh the following day and as many times as you need. That is the beauty of IF.

Minimized but conscious effort can bring about 80% of your significant changes. Such minimal but effective practices would be 5 minutes of HIIT, strength training, dance or squats. Do them three days a week. It is also essential to check your calcium absorption for efficient body functioning. To increase calcium metabolism, intake the right amount of vitamin D, K_2, and magnesium. You can also boost calcium absorption with exotic soup recipes like green and grain, beans, bone marrow, and fish. Finally, take the 7-day challenge to push your limits and redefine your boundaries. Oi, it is only 7 days.

But you'll feel so great that you will rinse and repeat.

7

FEASTING FORMULA

There is more to this formula than just eating the right amount of the right things. There are many whens, hows and whys to explore so that you start seeing results! Here, I will help you choose the right combination.

Eating Order

First, let me share a prescribed formula for consuming food that is beneficial to prevent blood sugar spikes, cravings, binging, and overeating, keep insulin and other hormones in check, and promote satiety so you stay fuller for longer. It's simple to follow when you know how.

School hours were 09:00hrs – 15:00hrs. We ate breakfast at home. During school hours, we enjoyed three breaks. A break before lunch, lunchtime at noon – 13:00, and another recess before school dismissed. We took a sandwich, some fruit, and sometimes a sweet or savory snack for packed lunch. It was not because of discipline that we did not eat during the break times. As children, it was our time to play and run around. We ate our meal at lunchtime, whether we brought it from home or bought it at school, including snacks. The next meal was at dinner time. We consumed our meals from around 07:30/08:00hrs to 16:00/20:00hrs. That was an 8–12-hour window of 3 meals depending on our parents' schedules. We were not into snacking, so we snacked or ate at another unplanned time, only occasionally. Fast forward to today, now that we leave home, we start eating erratically, all day into all night hours until bedtime, which causes excess inflammation. Plus, we get too busy to exercise or even too mature to play.

To iterate, let's get back to basics. Start with your childhood twelve-hour eating window, next extend to 10 and then 8 hours. Eating within an 8-hour window means eating 80% healthily and 20% treats. Refrain from overeating but don't skimp on your meals. Eat big meals and have higher protein in your last meal to keep you satisfied for longer.

While intermittent fasting, consuming any caloric food or beverage breaks the fast. You are allowed to enjoy your snacks during your eating window.

While you may still lose weight, skipping all indulgent foods during your fasting window is best to achieve all the benefits of autophagy. These include vitamins, supplements, non-caloric flavored drinks, non-caloric sweeteners, sugar-free gum and mints, essential oil, lemon, lime, apple cider vinegar, milk, and cream. I also abstain from bone broth, soup, sugar, honey, coconut oil, MCT, butter, BCAA, energy drinks, and protein meal replacement shakes. Feel free to grab them during the eating window.

Drink water and non-fruit herbal teas such as cinnamon, mint, ginger, chamomile and more. I mostly brew loose teas. Your fasting liquids may also comprise water with salt, electrolytes, black coffee, and black or green tea. Vitamins, supplements, and probiotics absorb best with meals. Consult your doctor for personalized advice especially addressing prescribed medication.

Meal Schedule

Three meals per day are for women who work hard physically or during menstruation, for ladies in peri-menopause or who have low blood sugar and crave sweets. It complements a simple breakfast, substantial lunch, and a small dinner that contains the most protein. It fits an easy intermittent schedule with an eating window between 08:00-18:00hrs and 14 hours of fasting.

Two meals per day help women develop good physical and mental qualities. This beginner level is suitable for the work week, with an eating window between noon-18:00hrs and 18 hours of fasting. Healthy snacks eaten within the eating window include rice cakes, carrot sticks, bee pollen, and microalgae: a substantial lunch and small dinner containing the most protein.

One meal per day is for women with firm discipline, supporting advanced development of mind and spirit. Fortunately, many women are sticking to the early time-restricted eating window between 11:00 – 13:00hrs trumping the intermediate level.

LEVELS UP:

- At the advanced level, women are water fasting once and twice weekly.
- And the veteran level is where women are water fasting every other day, three times per week—Mondays, Wednesdays, and Fridays.

The hours and days are adjustable to lifestyle and social preferences.

Difficulty Level	Meals	Eating Window	Fasting Hours
Easy	3 meals per day	08:00 -18:00 hours	14 hours
Beginner	2 meals per day	12:00 -18:00 hours	18 hours
Intermediate	1 meals per day	11:00 – 13:00 hours	20 - 22 hours
Advanced	Water fast	-	Once or twice weekly, example, Tuesday and Thursday
Veteran	Water fast	-	Every other day, example, Monday, Wednesday, and Friday

35% grains, 25% vegetables including sea vegetables, 15% legumes, 10% animal products, 8% nuts and oil-rich seeds, and 2% fruits is the proportion of food eaten in populations where women live longer and more robustly and experience less heart disease and cancer. Accordingly, consuming a harmonized diet of whole grains, vegetables, fruits, and the right fats and protein makes women melt excess fat rapidly because a low-carb and low-protein diet burns calories faster. Conversely, refined carbohydrates, white bread, sugar, pasta, pastries, fast and fried foods, and intoxicants cause demineralization and loss of nutrients and minerals, including magnesium.

Food Combination Formula

Kiss: Keep It Simply Simple to achieve digestive excellence.

Macronutrients are fats, proteins and carbohydrates. They split into three categories of food: acidic, alkaline, and neutral. Proteins such as meats, fowl, fish, eggs, yogurt, cheese, dried beans, and lentils are acidic; starches such as grains and their sprouts, bread, pasta, potatoes, sweet potatoes, beets, pumpkins, and squashes are alkaline; and fats and oils, and leafy green are neutral.

Eat the same few meals but plan each meal to contain different ingredients from the last and wait 4 hours between meals.

Eat the most protein-dense foods first because they require more stomach acids than other foods – nuts, seeds, and animal products.

Otherwise, left until last, there would not be enough stomach acids remaining to digest proteins.

Eat savory foods before other flavors. The best way is to combine salt at the beginning of the meal; for example, legumes which are proteins, are prepared with more salt; therefore, it is best to eat them before grains. Make use of the savory soups in Chapter 6 as meal starters.

Combine protein, fats, and starches with or at the same time as greens and non-starchy vegetables. Eat proteins with generous amounts of vitamin-enriched green vegetables such as leafy greens, cabbages, asparagus, alfalfa, green beans, zucchini, and seaweed. Accordingly, increase the intake of vital micronutrients into the body.

For easy digestion, combine proteins with starchy vegetables in a ratio of one to seven, for example, beans to grains. This combination helps avoid eating excess animal protein altogether. Cultures with high-protein diets have elevated levels of heart disease and osteoporosis.

Additionally, an allocation of protein, especially from animal products to starchy vegetables in a two-to-one ratio, is the cause of indigestion and inflammation because animal products are already rich in saturated fats and then usually fried in oil. Fats and oils significantly retard the digestion of proteins. In addition, excess fatty and oily foods ruin the liver. Pair your starchy snack with protein in a seven-to-one ratio by topping your banana chips with almond butter, and go easy on the nachos with cheese. Add chia seeds to add fiber to your snacks.

It is best to have a single starch in a meal, although the stomach may tolerate two types of starch because each type requires a different environment to digest well.

High-fat proteins, fats, and oils combine best with non-starchy green vegetables and sour, acidic fruits, for example, yogurt with strawberries, cottage cheese with grapefruits, almonds and tart apples, whole sesame butter with lemon sauce, and turkey and cranberry sauce. For this reason, a high-fat protein salad of nuts, seeds, avocado, olives, or yogurt combines well with the acidic fruits of lemons, limes, and tomatoes. These tart fruits also combine well with green and low-starch vegetables. For example, Greek salad consists of creamy Greek feta cheese blocks, olive oil, tomatoes, olives, cucumbers, bell peppers, and red onions.

Acids, when combined with proteins before cooking, break down the protein chains and make fats more digestible, for example, marinating meat with vinegar and then cooking them. Nevertheless, when eaten after protein, acids stop the stomach from completely digesting proteins because they prevent the stomach from secreting digestive acids.

Fats and oils consist of little protein. Fats are avocados, olives, butter, cream, and sour cream; oils are olive oil, coconut oil, sesame oil, flax oil, and ghee. They do not retard the digestion of starch which is why bread and butter, bread and avocado, rice and olives, and cream and flax oil over oatmeal combine deliciously well. Fats and oil digest well with green vegetables. They also digest well in starchy meals with lots of green vegetables.

Another combination is with acidic fruits, as in an oil and lemon juice salad dressing.

Eating fruits and sweetened food separately from other foods is best for optimal digestion. Since they are better on an empty stomach, the first meal of the day consisting of only fruit and fruit juices with their fiber has a desirable cleansing effect on the digestive system as it eliminates the fermentation caused by poor food combination and excess meat.

When combined with a meal, eating fruits and sweetened food in small quantities at the end of the meal is preferable because they do not mix well with proteins and starches. Drink fruit juices in their pulp no less than 4 hours after a protein meal and 2 hours after a starchy meal. The simple carbohydrate structure of fruits, such as melons and concentrated sweeteners, cause them to digest first, leaving other foods to ferment and not digest properly. However, green vegetables such as lettuce and celery enhance the digestion of fruits and simple sugars and eliminate inflammation from any fermenting foods in the digestive system.

When you eat fruits in the wrong order in a meal, the fruits digest first and make the other foods, such as protein and starchy and green vegetables, wait to be digested. The waiting causes this food to ferment in the gut. Fermentation builds excess inflammation. Celery and lettuce help to reduce damp conditions such as inflammation in the stomach.

So, save the best for the last and have your sweet after you finish your lunch or dinner, followed by lettuce or celery sticks. Healthy sweets include raisins, 1/2 oz square of 86% dark chocolate, dates, baked sweet potato, sweet potato chips, apple chips, fresh or frozen fruits like grapes, and homemade smoothies.

Celery contains cancer-fighting components like flavonoids, phthalides, and polyacetylenes. An anti-inflammatory consisting of luteolin and pyrroloquinoline quinone PQQ, celery reduces stress hormones and treats constipation. It also contains powerful electrolytes that aid the nervous system. For example, luteolin boosts the T3 hormone in the thyroid. As an antiseptic, it eliminates urinary tract infections and kidney and bladder disorders. It also improves memory and supports heart health, digestive function, and blood sugar management.

After sweet desserts like ice cream and cake, eat celery sticks to stop your craving for sweets on its track. Fresh celery sticks contain fiber which benefits weight maintenance and reduces low-density lipids (LDL), the bad cholesterol. But first, consult your doctor if you have a sensitive digestive system like irritable bowel syndrome (IBS) and allergic reactions such as skin rashes and anaphylaxis.

Do not drink milk with other foods. Milk ferments around any foods you eat it with and stops them from being digested. The exception is that the already fermented milk combines well with green vegetables like buttermilk, yogurt, and cheese.

The following order and meal combination are optimal:

1. Proteins
2. Vegetables/fats
3. Starches

4. Fruit/dessert
5. Large lettuce salad/celery sticks

Food Combinations To Acknowledge

Just like eating order is essential, so are food combinations. Mixing and matching different types of foods can make your digestive system work harder, resulting in poor digestion. Keeping it straightforward, here are some food combinations to avoid:

- Avoid eating sweet fruits with acidic fruits like pomegranates with oranges.
- Avoid mixing mucus-forming foods, eggs and dairy with a grain-based diet to prevent excess inflammation and constipation.
- Avoid drinking too much liquid with meals except for warm water and ACV in small quantities.
- Do not combine different types of protein in the same meal.
- Avoid consuming fats and proteins together.
- Avoid eating fruits alongside grains like wheat, barley, and rice.
- Do not combine hot drinks with mangoes, meat, dairy, or fish.

Here are some food combinations to apply:

- Eat the highest protein-dense foods in the meal first.
- Eat savory foods before other flavors.
- Pair green and non-starchy vegetables with proteins, fats, and starches.
- Fats and oils combine well with starches.
- Fats and oils digest well with green vegetables.
- Fats and oils with starchy meals digest best with plenty of leafy green vegetables.

- High-fat proteins – nuts, oil-rich seeds, and fermented dairy foods – cheese, yogurt, and kefir are a good combination with acidic fruits.
- Acidic fruits: Lemon, lime, and tomato are good combinations with green and non-starchy vegetables.
- Eat fruits on their own.
- For dessert, eat small quantities of fruits and sweet foods at the end of the meal.
- Lettuce and celery are a good combination with all fruits. Eat them after a fruit dessert and sweetened food.
- Drink milk separately from other foods.

As important as determining what to eat and when to eat, it is equally important to evaluate the correct eating order. By eating foods in the recommended sequence, you can expect greater mental clarity, weight loss, a significant reduction in insulin levels, improved digestive health, and even better sleep quality! Eating each meal like a three-course meal in a restaurant is satiating. After sweet desserts like ice cream and cake, eat celery sticks to stop the sweet craving on its track.

8

CONSCIOUS CELEBRATION

Step 3

"Come on! Take a cheat day! You've earned it." Your well-meaning friends may be well-meaning, but taking that excessive cheat day could be your undoing. I'm not saying you can't have the occasional ice cream treat; I'm just saying there are better and healthier alternatives to rewarding yourself for a job well done! Because they will be many. Ask yourself, is it a 'nice to have' or a 'must have'? While movies and tv shows may show stick-thin models gouging out on their cheat days, real-life requires much more effort. We shall look at ways you can reach your worthy goal and celebrate each win. We don't want two steps ahead and one step backward. We want one step front, another step forward, and so on. So, let's look at how you can cultivate this conscious celebration.

Intuitive Awareness

For whom are you implementing this lifestyle change? For whom are you eating healthy? Your doctor who nags you every time you visit? Your daughter who berates you for being unhealthy every chance she gets? Your husband - no, not him. You understand your body best, so you know what you need, Boss. Develop a fitness plan that fits you best, and do it yourself! The first step to finding inspiration is finding it within yourself. Only then will you truly be able to persevere toward your goal. Even if you don't like fasting, as you continue doing it, you will realize you do it because you desire how it feels when you lose those extra pounds. Even if you don't like eating your leafy greens, you'll start eating them for how much you like your regular bowel movements and healthy gut. You will have made the process yours.

Increased Financial Gain

If you're not satiating every craving, here is a fun fact: your wallet will be much fuller than before! This formula not only teaches you self-restraint and self-control but also allows you to look within yourself and question what you need and don't need in life. Not only will you eat out less, but you will also consciously adhere to previously incomplete lifestyle decisions. You have a plan to stick to, making your life much more disciplined and planned. You'll find that you have freed up finances for your spontaneous urges. Win-Win!

Physical Rewards

You will notice your body is light and airy once you lose those extra pounds. You will soon be testifying: "I eat mindfully and am in control of food. My stomach feels better due to cutting off eating time because I do not eat until bedtime. I now sleep peacefully and soundly. I am more energetic. I release weight easily and see myself achieving my ideal weight and staying there. I am achieving perfect health. I found my miracle pill to stop overeating, binge eating, and addiction indulgence." And this is all true!

Psychological Stimulation

Now that you have put mind over matter, you will have more cognitive clarity. You are the winner! You did it! With such a positive mindset, you slowly built much-needed positive self-esteem. You are now in control of your body, and while getting to this point, you have become unbreakable, you stuck it out and did what you had to do, and you made it! You got rid of all the negative notions of ageing, like 'gaining weight is inevitable,' 'the body deteriorates with age,' and 'you cannot do anything about it.'

Tracking

Remember how I asked you to measure yourself in the beginning? First, take a few pictures to track how far you've come. Then, whip out the consistent measuring tool and measure yourself. Now that you are reassessing yourself, see how all your hard work has paid off. Nothing is more satisfying than seeing the fruit of your labour. You no longer enviously watch other women's social media before and after videos. You have successfully conquered the before and after!

Another part of tracking how far you've come is keeping a journal to write about your achievements appreciatively. Having a grateful heart and understanding that while you did the heavy lifting, being thankful to your family who has stood by you as you maintained this strict or semi-flexible window and your friends who encouraged you on days you wanted to quit. And, of course, God, who kept you healthy throughout this process and provided you with all you needed, is essential. So, pen your gratitude and see how many people, circumstances, things, and events are for you.

Another good way of tracking your achievements is by seeking at least five peers on this weight release journey and tracking achievements with them. Not to say this is a competition of any sort, but it is a good motivator when you need that little push.

Celebrate Wins Exuberantly

You did it! You deserve a celebration. Depending on your personality type, you will celebrate alone or with your loved ones and engage in activities that bring you the most joy. Rather than taking the easy route and scoffing down ten chocolate bars or whipping out the barbeque grill, don't kid yourself. Initiate alternatives to celebrating this authentic achievement. Some suggestions:

Focus on the positives and write them in your gratefulness journal with the dates. You know how the song goes:

"Count your blessings, name them one by one, count your blessings, see what God has done, and it will surprise you what the LORD has done!"

We tend to overlook so much, but by organizing your thoughts, you will see how much there is to be grateful.

- A scented candle bath: You can't go wrong with a long, warm magnesium bath with a scented candle. Let the sensations take you away.
- Candle-lit dinner with a lover or loved ones: You can eat! Just be sure not to go crazy with processed meat or alcohol.
- Cuddles: With your favorite person? With your pet? The world is your oyster.
- A massage: There is nothing a good massage can't fix. My go-to if I want to reward myself for a well-and-dusted job.
- A mani-pedi: It's always a good time, so book an appointment and treat yourself.
- A sauna treatment: will be a lovely and relaxing time for your body and skin.
- Physical recreation: This relaxation mode is separate from exercise! You could go out and get your body moving in a way you can enjoy! Go to your local park and sleep in the sun.
- Or go to the zoo. I bet you haven't been in a while.

- An amusement park with your family is your idea of a fun time. Yes, I love a screaming adventure. A nature trek is always lovely, and the views are always rewarding.
- Or you could finally take that long-overdue vacation to Hawaii.

You could build these celebrations into your daily, weekly, or monthly routine. They will make the IF process fun, be incredible motivators, and provide psychological ascension.

A win is a win, no matter how small or big. By learning to appreciate your wins, you'll end up motivating yourself in ways you wouldn't have been able to if you'd just brushed them off as small events. The fact is motivation plays a huge role in determining whether you succeed or fail. So, who will stop you if you can reward yourself and celebrate the small wins? Press on to find out how you can celebrate small successes:

REWARD yourself

As simple as it gets. Use one of the above-given tips or indulge in a hobby. You've earned it.

BREAK DOWN significant goals into smaller milestones

By doing so, you're creating pitstops for yourself. So, you can survey how far you've come at every juncture and appreciate the journey, as each small step will progress to the big goal.

DO NOT PUT TOO much pressure on yourself

Cracking under pressure is the last thing you need. Putting too much pressure on yourself will result in the opposite, with your pushing your body too far and raising cortisol levels. Be aware of your limits and stick to them. Take baby steps. Every day may not deliver a new achievement, but that makes the eventual triumphs much sweeter.

TRACK **your progress**

By doing so, you can know which wins you are celebrating. So, get tracking!

Change your perspective on life and yourself: Instead of looking at a distant mountain, surpass the roads and the slopes right ahead. That will make your goals a lot more realistic to realize.

Yayy! You are on the other side of the bridge. You have survived the stomach-wrenching journey, and caution: Consciously! Did you notice that on this IF journey, you developed intuitive awareness? Don't hold back. Keep tracking and keep winning. Start journaling how much fat you melt using the formula and all your non-scale-victories. And if you have not guessed yet, the third and final step is celebrating. Celebrate big, small and all victories! Dance with me, "Celebrate good times. Come On!"

Give other women in their 50s and beyond the chance to lose stubborn fat and be their best, most energized selves.

You now know how to make intermittent fasting your best ally, and you have seen how this simple, easy-to-implement system has enabled you to lose stubborn fat in less than 27 days.

Simply by leaving your honest opinion of this book on Amazon, you'll help other women look and feel better than they have in years. Chronic disease and obesity are not something women should accept as a normal part of aging.

WANT TO HELP OTHERS?

Thank you for being so helpful. You can help other women harmonize their hormones, boost their 12 body systems, and stay motivated to look and feel better than they were in their 40s.

More Empowerment To You

I can't believe I am writing the conclusion already. I was still determining where I was heading when writing this book. I didn't even know I would write a book on intermittent fasting. I mean, picture this, a woman in her 50s who has always struggled with an array of health issues, obesity, and mobility restrictions, to name a few, will end up writing a book on health that talks about shedding those stubborn pounds with no rigorous exercises and diet regime.

I know, fantastic, but this is how it ended up happening. When I started my IF journey, I had zero expectations. Almost convinced it was just another fad that won't budge my fat. But I was astonished, amazed, and taken aback. Thankfully. And I was itching to share my story.

Initially, even if I had helped a single woman to take on IF and shed a few pounds, I would have considered myself successful. However, my journey has ignited the hidden spark within countable women. Countable because I don't want to make bold claims. Claims never take you anywhere. Proactive steps, aggressive mindsets, and fierce beliefs do. You are already halfway there if you have already pictured yourself in that cute little black dress, irrespective of age. It all starts in your head.

To recap, I talked about my journey, how useless a chunk of fat I used to be, and how I transformed myself into a graceful lady. Why twenty-seven days? After doing the same thing for twenty-one days, three weeks, you form a habit. *News Break: while it takes 21 days to change your mind, it takes 40 days to break addictions and concrete any change.* Inch by inch, every pound shed is a cinch.

It takes one step to get started, use the information from this book that resonates with you, and repeat. You'll observe notable changes, your once-tight clothes fitting loosely, and the rewards encourage you to continue. Finally, as the days draw to the twenty-seventh day, your body exclaims, this is working. Your measurements show your weight taking a nosedive. Eventually, this caterpillar evacuates her chrysalis, and you become a bold and beautiful butterfly. You are lovely and light, and there is no stopping you. Your new life has begun!

I propose two simple steps to fast intermittently – determine when and what to eat. That's all. That's all it takes to practice IF. 'What' ensures that you don't make your bodily systems overwork, and 'when' ensures that your physical systems get to rest. The result? Optimum body function. I can't stop comparing this to a machine; that's what we are: a biological machine.

Intermittent fasting doesn't just help you melt fat, but it overhauls your entire lifestyle. When was the last time you fasted? I had never fasted when I first started this journey. Imagine you are making your digestive system work 24/7 without any rest. And not just work, but overwork, all thanks to the junk, fat, grease, and chemicals we put in our body as if it were a trash can. Isn't it customary that it will start acting up one day? Even machines do.

And then the entire system starts getting messed up and noisy. Hormones scream, your sleeping schedule gets disturbed, your monthly cycle gets obstructed, and the list is endless. But, of course, you already know what I am discussing now.

Even if you are in the best shape, I recommend intermittent fasting a few days a week. Nevertheless, putting your weight loss journey aside, if you want to add rejuvenation and vigor to your life, this is one action we all must engage in for stamina. But, of course, pay attention to spiritual fulfilment, quality sleep, synergistic relationships, stress management and easy exercise. The way I see it, all of these are the by-products of a healthy lifestyle that starts with eating the right things at the right time.

I know all it takes is two simple steps, but there is one still more to it - CELEBRATION! So first, look at yourself in the mirror and give yourself a flying kiss. Then, pat your back, and celebrate. You did well, darling!

Adding to the bargain, I also included a few of my favorite Mediterranean recipes to please your taste buds in exuberance and as nutritiously as possible. Finally, for Indian food lovers, you will also find some lip-smacking Indian recipes towards the end.

This book has been my sincere endeavor to spring consciousness into our eating habits so we are not straining our bodies. Still, we are pursuing a holistic formula that enriches it from the inside rather than just satiating our taste buds.

I invite you to continue this expedition; you won't regret it. This passage will help you push doors, redefine your boundaries, establish a better connection with your body and establish the freedom to live a healthy, productive life.

I am cheering for you and will run to embrace you on the other side of this bridge. Cheers to your joyful existence!

9

BONUS: MEDITERRANEAN RECIPES

Whether vegan, vegetarian, pescatarian, omnivore, or carnitarian, in addition to the calcium-absorption soups in Chapter 6, here are recipes to meet your dietary requirement. As promised, let's explore the best Mediterranean recipes.

ROASTED VEGETABLES with Green Salsa
Serves people: 4
415 cals per serving
Preparation time: 40 minutes
Cooking time: 50 minutes
Ingredients:

- 2 small aubergines (eggplants)
- 2 zucchinis (courgettes)
- 1 yellow bell pepper
- 1 red bell pepper
- 8 cloves of garlic
- 90 ml (6 tbsp) extra-virgin olive oil

- 15 ml (1 tbsp) Italian herbs
- 6 ripe plum tomatoes, quartered
- 60 ml (4 tbsp) chopped fresh parsley
- 30 ml (2 tbsp) chopped fresh mint
- 2 cloves garlic, peeled and crushed
- 1 red chili pepper, deseeded
- 5 ml (1 tsp) Dijon mustard
- 7.5 ml (1 ½ tsp) lemon juice
- 120 ml (4 Fl oz) cold-pressed extra-virgin olive oil
- Celtic salt
- Pepper

Instructions:

- Prepare green salsa by placing parsley, mint, garlic, red chili pepper, Dijon mustard, lemon juice, and 120 ml oil in a food processor and process until smooth and season with salt and pepper to taste.
- Transfer the mix to a bowl and set aside to infuse.
- Cut the aubergines (eggplants) lengthways into thick slices of 5 mm (½ cm).
- Place them on a lightly oiled large baking sheet.
- Cut the zucchinis (courgettes) into 1.27 cm (½ inch) slices.
- Deseed the peppers and cut them into thin strips.
- Transfer the zucchinis (courgettes), peppers, and unpeeled garlic cloves to a large roasting tin. Mix 90 ml oil with herbs and drizzle half over the vegetables.
- Brush the aubergine (eggplant) slices with herb-flavored oil.
- Place the roasting tin containing the zucchinis (courgettes), garlic, and peppers on the top shelf of the oven at 230°C (450°F) mark 8, with the aubergines (eggplants) on the second shelf for half an hour.
- Add the tomatoes to the roasting tin containing the zucchinis (courgettes), peppers and garlic and stir well.

Turn the aubergine (eggplant) slices and brush with the remaining herb-flavored oil. Return the roasting tin containing the aubergines (eggplants) to the oven. Cook for a further 10 - 20 minutes until tender. Let it stand for three minutes.
- Drizzle green salsa.
- Serve hot.

Mediterranean Egg Plants
Serves people: 4
344 cals per serving
Preparation time: 15 minutes
Cooking time: 20 minutes
Ingredients:

- 60 ml (4 tbsp) extra-virgin olive oil
- 1 ½ large yellow onions, halved and sliced
- 30 ml (2 tbsp) vegetable broth or white wine.
- ⅓ cup firmly packed julienne-cut sun-dried tomatoes
- 1 clove of garlic, minced
- 1 large aubergine (eggplant) stem removed and cut breadthways into 5 mm (½ cm) thick slices
- 3 ounces crumbled feta cheese (vegan feta optional)
- Celtic salt
- Freshly ground black pepper
- Parsley, finely chopped

Instructions:

- Heat the oil on medium heat in a large stainless-steel skillet.
- Toss onions into the pan and stir gently to coat them evenly in the oil. For about two minutes, keep stirring until they are soft and attain a deep brown color.

- Add the vegetable broth or white wine to the pan and stir, allowing the broth to cook off and pick up all the caramelized bits at the bottom of the pan.
- Add garlic and sun-dried tomatoes and cook for about three minutes or until fragrant.
- Arrange the mixture in an even layer in the pan, then carefully place the aubergines (eggplants) over the top. Sprinkle it with crumbled feta cheese, Celtic salt, and pepper.
- Cook for 10 minutes, covered with a tight-fitting lid.
- Remove pan from heat and sprinkle with chopped parsley.
- Serve hot.

Sardines with Herbs

Serves people: 4
570 cals per serving
Preparation time: 10 - 30 minutes
Cooking time: 10 minutes
Ingredients:

- 900 g (2 lb) 12 sardines, gutted
- 120 ml (4 Fl oz) olive oil
- 45 ml (3 tbsp) lemon juice
- 10 ml (2 tsp) grated lemon zest
- 60 ml (2 tbsp) chopped mixed herbs - parsley, thyme, chervil
- Celtic salt
- Pepper

Instructions:

- Mix oil, lemon juice, lemon zest, herbs, and seasoning in a bowl.

- Arrange the sardines on a grill rack, drizzle the herbs dressing over them, and grill for 5 - 7 minutes on each side, frequently basting with dressing.
- Serve hot or cold.

Main Course

Salmon Filets with Basil and Balsamic Vinegar

Serves people: 4
540 cals per serving
Preparation time: 30 minutes, plus marinating
Cooking time: 8 minutes
Ingredients:

- 4 Salmon filets, 170g (6 oz) each
- 30 ml (2 tbsp) balsamic vinegar
- 90 ml (6 tbsp) extra-virgin olive oil
- 40 g (1 ½ oz) fresh basil, stalks removed
- 8 ripe plum tomatoes, skinned, deseeded, and diced
- 30 ml (2 tbsp) chopped fresh chives.
- 4 clove garlic pressed and crushed.
- 1 lemon
- Celtic salt
- Pepper

Instructions:

- Clean salmon by descaling and washing them with lemon in water. Blend basil, olive oil, balsamic vinegar, salt, and pepper. Rub garlic onto the filets, then season with balsamic vinegar, basil, olive oil, salt, and pepper. Arrange the salmon filets in a shallow baking dish. Set aside to marinate for 30 minutes.

- Mix the tomatoes with the chives, and season well with salt, pepper, and olive oil in a bowl. Cover and leave to infuse.
- Preheat oven broiler.
- Broil the salmon for 15 minutes about 6 inches from the heat source, turning once, or until browned on both sides and easily flaked with a fork. Brush occasionally with the balsamic, basil, and olive oil sauce.
- Bake tomato chive mixture for 5 minutes.
- Whisk the balsamic, basil, and olive oil mixture to recombine.
- Spoon the tomato mixture onto the toasty serving plates and place salmon filets on top. Drizzle with the balsamic, basil, and olive oil mixture and garnish with basil.
- Lovely with asparagus spears.

Garlic and Rosemary Roast Leg of Lamb

Serves people: 8
290 cals per serving
Preparation time: 20 minutes
Cooking time: 3 hours
Ingredients:

- 2.7 kg (6 lb) leg of lamb
- 3 garlic cloves, peeled and cut into slivers
- Small bunch of fresh rosemary sprigs
- 30 ml (2 tbsp) smoked paprika
- 30 ml (2 tbsp) olive oil
- 150 ml (¼ pint) red wine
- 300 ml (½ pint) lamb stock
- Celtic Salt
- Pepper

Instructions:

- Slice shallow cuts into the fatty white layer of the lamb and create diamond shapes. Massage the lamb with a drizzle of olive oil, then season with salt, plenty of pepper, and paprika.
- Make incisions over the meat and deeply insert a tiny sprig of rosemary and a sliver of garlic into each slit.
- Let it marinate for 2 hours.
- Place in a roasting tin and roast at 230ºC (450ºF) mark 8 for 15 minutes. Lower the setting to 200ºC (400ºF) mark 6 and cook for 2 hours, basting occasionally.
- Lift the lamb onto a warmed serving platter and put it to rest in a warm place for 10 minutes.
- Drain the fat from the tin into a pot and add red wine and stock to make gravy. Boil to reduce and then strain into a sauce boat. Add salt and pepper to taste.
- After carving the lamb, serve it with gravy.
- Serve with warm roasted vegetable salad.

Chicken Breast Stuffed with Mushrooms

Serves people: 6
500 cals per serving
Preparation time: 25 minutes
Cooking time: 30 minutes
Ingredients:

- 30 ml (2 tbsp) olive oil
- 2 shallots, peeled and finely chopped
- 45 ml (3 tbsp) chopped parsley
- 45 ml (3 tbsp) Italian seasoning
- 125 g (4 oz) ghee
- 30 ml (2 tbsp) chopped basil
- A squeeze of lemon juice
- 6 chicken breast filets with skin
- Wooden skewers or toothpicks
- Cooking string or twine

- Celtic Salt
- Pepper

Instructions:

- Season chicken filets with salt, pepper, and Italian herbs, and let them marinate.
- Heat the olive oil on a heavy-based frying pan to make the mushroom stuffing. Add the shallot and gently cook until softened but not browned. Add the mushrooms and continue cooking until well reduced and softened. Remove from heat.
- To make the herb ghee, heat 75 g (3 oz) until soft, then add the parsley, basil, lemon juice, and a pinch of salt and pepper. Transfer to a small baking tin and place in the refrigerator. Chill until firm.
- When the mushroom stuffing is cold, carefully loosen the skin from each chicken breast, keeping it attached along one side. Cut the chicken breast in half lengthways. Spoon the mushroom stuffing into the chicken slit.
- Secure the stuffing by pushing a fine wooden skewer through the skin, using toothpicks, and tying the chicken into a neat parcel with string.
- Lay the chicken in a roasting tin, with the stuffed side upwards.
- Melt the remaining ghee and brush over the chicken. Roast at (200ºC (400ºF) mark 6 for 30 minutes until cooked straight through.
- Cut the herb ghee into slices. Transfer the chicken breasts to a toasty serving platter and top with a couple of slices of herb ghee. Serve immediately. Serve with bok choy.

Walnut Roasted Beef Steaks
Serves people: 6
750 cals per serving

Preparation time: 30 minutes plus cooling
Cooking time: 20 minutes
Ingredients:

- 1.1kg (2 ½ lb) piece filet of beef, trimmed
- 45 ml (3 tbsp) avocado oil. 60 ml (4 tbsp) white wine
- 300 ml (½ pint) beef stock
- 5 ml (1 tsp) gravy browning
- 350 g (12 oz) walnut pieces, roughly chopped
- 125 g (4 oz) pickled walnuts, drained and chopped
- 50 g (2 oz) can anchovies, drained
- 5 cloves of garlic, peeled
- Celtic salt and pepper
- 60 ml (4 tbsp) chopped fresh parsley

Instructions:

- Mix the roughly chopped walnut and pickled walnuts to prepare the walnut paste. Set half aside. Put the other half in the blender and process with the anchovies, garlic, and olive oil until smooth. Add the other half of the walnuts with Celtic salt and pepper, and stir to achieve a thick, clumpy paste.
- With a sharp knife, slice the filet into six thick steaks. In a heavy-based frying pan, heat the oil until almost smoking. Fry the steaks quickly on each side to brown and seal. Allow cooling. Top each steak thickly with the walnut paste. Cover and refrigerate until ready to cook.
- To allow the steak to come to room temperature, remove them from the refrigerator 20 minutes before cooking.
- Place the steaks on a baking sheet. Bake in the oven at 200ºC (400ºF) mark 6 for 15 minutes, depending on thickness and preferred cooking finish.
- Make the gravy: Place the frying pan used to fry the steak on the hob over medium heat and deglaze it with the

wine, stirring to scrape up the sediments. Add the beef stock and gravy browning. Bring to a boisterous boil and allow to bubble for 2 - 3 minutes until slightly reduced. Pour into a warm gravy boat.
- Serve the steaks as soon as they are cooked with plenty of freshly chopped parsley and accompanied by gravy.

Fruity Stuffed Roasted Turkey
Serves people: 15
350 cals per serving
Preparation time: 20 minutes
Cooking time: 3 ½ hours, plus resting time
Ingredients:

- 1 oven-ready turkey with giblets of about 4.5 kg (10 lb)
- 90 ml (6 tbsp) avocado oil
- 60 ml (4 tbsp) chopped fresh parsley
- 20 ml (4 tsp) chopped fresh rosemary
- 1 whole sprig of rosemary
- 15 ml (1 tbsp) dry oregano leaves
- 5 ml (1 tsp) crushed red chili flakes
- 200 g (3 ½ oz) onion, peeled and roughly chopped
- 200 g (7 oz) mushrooms, roughly chopped
- 125 g (4 oz) celery, finely sliced
- 125 g (4 oz) ready-to-eat dried apricots, finely chopped
- 15 ml (1 tbsp) chopped fresh sage
- 1.25 ml (¼ tbs) dried Italian spice
- 15 ml Dijon mustard
- Celtic salt
- Pepper

For the gravy:

- 570 ml (1.2 pints) chicken stock
- 300 ml (10.14 Fl oz) dry apple cider

- 4 roughly chopped garlic cloves
- 3 roughly chopped tomatoes
- 2 sprigs of rosemary.
- 1 roughly chopped onion
- Metal skewers.

Instructions:

- Treat the turkey: Remove the neck and giblets from cavities. Rinse turkey thoroughly with cold water, drain, and pat dry with paper towels. Tuck wing tips under the back or tie them to the body. Loosen the skin at the neck end of the turkey, loosening the skin on the breast using your fingers. With a small knife, remove the wishbone.
- Combine parsley, rosemary, oregano, red chili flakes, salt, and pepper with 60 ml avocado oil and apply this combination to the skin. Leave to marinate.
- Make the stuffing: Heat the remaining 30 ml avocado oil in a frying pan, add the onions, and gently fry for 5 minutes. Add celery and mushroom and briskly fry for 5 minutes. Add the apricots, pistachio nuts, Dijon mustard, sage, and Italian spice with fried celery and mushroom into a bowl. Season with Celtic salt and pepper. Stir well and allow to cool.
- Spoon the stuffing into the turkey, then shape it neatly. Tuck the neck skin under and secure it with metal skewers —Refasten drumsticks with metal clips or a band of skin.
- Place the turkey in a roasting tin, breast side down, and spread with oil. Place the giblets and lemon halves around the turkey, then cover with foil to make a tent.
- Roast the turkey: Roast in the oven at 190°C (375°F) mark 5, basting regularly. Circa 45 minutes before the end of cooking time, remove the foil, turn the turkey over and continue baking until the juices run clear. Inject a skewer into the thickest part of the thigh to ensure the juices run

- clear. Carefully tilt the bird to allow the juices in the cavity to run into the tin. Relocate the turkey to a warm toasty platter, cover it with foil and leave it to rest in a warm place for 2.5 hours or for the same duration as baking time, covered with foil and towel.
- Make the gravy: Skim most of the roasting tin fat, leaving about 30 ml (2 tbsp) of fat. Add the giblets. Place over medium heat. Add chopped onions, garlic, rosemary sprigs, roasted lemon, and tomatoes. Stir and cook for 1 minute. Add the dry apple cider and bubble for 1 minute. As the cider reduces, pour in the meat juices, including juice from the rested turkey. After reducing the liquid by half, crush the ingredients with a masher. Next, pour in the chicken stock. Bring back to boil and bubble for 10 minutes to reduce by about half to thicken it. Add a sprig of rosemary to infuse for 1 minute. Skim off any fat and sieve. Serve in a warmed gravy boat.
- Carve the turkey into slices and serve with the stuffing, accompaniments, gravy, and vegetables.

Chili Black Beans

Serves people: 3
382 cals per serving
Preparation time: 12 hours
Cooking time: 75 minutes
Ingredients:

- 400 g dried black beans
- 400 g cherry tomatoes
- 1 large orange bell pepper, deseeded and diced
- 1 large red onion, halved and sliced
- 2 garlic cloves, sliced
- 15 ml (3 tsp) tomato paste
- 10 ml (2 tsp) chili powder
- 5 ml (1 tsp) ground cumin

- 5 ml (1 tsp) paprika
- 300 ml (½ pint) vegetable stock
- 30 ml (2 tbsp) extra-virgin olive oil
- Celtic salt

Instructions:

- Clean the beans: Arrange the beans in a single layer and remove any visible debris. Wash off grit by placing the beans in a colander and running cold water through them.
- In a pot, cover the beans with 2 inches of water. Add two tablespoons of Celtic salt and allow them to soak for 12 hours or overnight. Drain and rinse before cooking.
- Place on low heat and stir occasionally. Cook for 45 to 60 minutes. Check that the beans are cooked by mashing them to ensure they are soft.
- To make chili beans, stir-fry the onions, garlic, and peppers in a pan until softened. Add the chili powder, ground cumin, paprika, and tomato paste, then pour in the vegetable stock. Stir in the tomatoes and cooked black beans. Cover and cook for 10 minutes. 6. Serve on a hot platter.

Spiced Lentils

Serves people: 3
392 cals per serving
Preparation time: 10 minutes
Cooking time: 30 minutes
Ingredients:

- 237 ml (1 cup) dried green lentils, cleaned and drained
- 1 large red onion, halved and sliced
- 4 cloves of garlic, sliced.
- 3 cups vegetable stock
- 3 cups baby spinach, washed and cleaned

- 2 large carrots, washed, peeled, and diced
- 1 large red bell pepper deseeded and chopped into medium squares to match diced carrots.
- 15 ml (3 tsp) dried basil
- 15 ml (3 tsp) dried oregano
- 10 ml (2 tsp) dried parsley
- 5 ml (1 tsp) ground sage
- 30 ml (2 tbsp) extra-virgin olive oil
- 10 ml (2 tsp) Celtic salt
- 10 ml (2 tsp) ground black pepper
- 2 bay leaves

Instructions:

- Clean the lentils: Arrange the lentils in a single layer on a sheet pan or kitchen towel and remove any visible debris. Wash the lentils properly in cold running water through a colander.
- Prepare the lentils: Transfer to a saucepan and add the vegetable stock and bay leaves. Over medium-high heat, after simmering briskly, reduce the heat for a soft simmer. Add stock to the narrowly opened pot and cook for 30 minutes. The cooking is complete when the lentils are tender. Strain the lentils and remove the bay leaves.
- Make spiced lentils: In a large pot, fry onions and garlic in olive oil until softened. Add basil, oregano, parsley, and sage. Pour in vegetable stock, lentils, and carrots and bring to a boil. Cover and let simmer for 10 minutes. Add bell peppers and simmer for 4 minutes. Add baby spinach, stir for 30 seconds, and remove from heat. Taste and add salt and ground pepper to taste.
- Serve while hot. Refrigerate for up to 4 days.

Asparagus Spears
Serves people: 4

145 cals per serving
Preparation time: 5 minutes
Ingredients:

- 20 asparagus spears
- 30 ml (2 tbsp) extra-virgin olive oil
- 100 ml (7 tbsp) nutritional yeast

Instructions:

- In boiling salted water, cook the asparagus for 4 mins.
- Drain, then toss with a bit of oil.
- Divide the asparagus between 4 plates and top each pile with nutritional yeast flakes.

Salads

Greek Salad
Serves people: 4
425 cals per serving
Preparation time: 15 minutes
Ingredients:

- 450 g (1 lb) ripe, flavorful tomatoes cut into chunks
- 1 cucumber, cut into chunks
- 1 large red onion, peeled and thinly sliced
- 75 g (3 oz) black olives
- 225 g (8 oz) creamy Greek feta cheese, cut into chunks

Dressing:

- 90 ml (6 tbsp) extra-virgin olive oil
- 30 ml (2 tbsp) lemon juice
- 1 garlic clove, peeled
- 45 ml (3 tbsp) chopped fresh oregano

- Celtic salt
- Pepper
- To garnish: chopped basil

Instructions:

- Combine the tomatoes, cucumber, and onion in a large bowl, then add the olives.
- To make the dressing, whisk the ingredients in a bowl or shake in a screw-topped jar until combined.
- Pour on the dressing and toss gently to mix. Scatter the feta cheese on top and serve, garnished with chopped basil.

Roasted Vegetable Salad
Serves people: 8
250 cals per serving
Preparation: 20 minutes, plus standing
Cooking time: 45 - 50 minutes
Ingredients:

- 2 aubergines
- 2 zucchinis
- 2 red peppers, halved, cored, and deseeded
- 2 small red onions, peeled and cut into wedges
- 1 fennel bulb, quartered, cored, and diced
- 15 ml (1 tbsp) chopped fresh thyme
- 15 ml (1 tbsp) chopped fresh sage
- 60 ml (4 tbsp) olive oil
- 1 small head of garlic
- 30 ml (2 tbsp) chopped fresh basil
- 25 g (1 oz) pitted black olives
- 25 g (1 oz) pine nuts, toasted
- Celtic salt
- Pepper

Dressing:

- 10 ml (2 tsp) balsamic or sherry vinegar
- 60 ml (4 tbsp) extra-virgin olive oil

Instructions:

- Cut the aubergines and zucchinis into cubes of 2.5 cm (1 inch). Layer in a colander, sprinkling with 10 ml (2 tsp) of Celtic salt. Set aside for 20 minutes, then rinse well to remove salt and dry on kitchen paper.
- Cut the peppers into 2.5 cm (1 inch) squares and place in a large bowl with the aubergines, zucchinis, onions, fennel, thyme, sage, and oil. Toss well, then place in a large roasting tin in a single layer or on several roasting tins.
- Slice the top from the head of the garlic and stand on a small sheet of foil. Drizzle oil, season, and seal the foil to form a parcel. Sit the parcel amongst the vegetables.
- Roast at 230ºC (450ºF) mark 8 for 45 - 50 minutes, occasionally stirring to ensure even browning. Transfer the vegetables to a large bowl.
- Unwrap the garlic and scoop the flesh into a bowl. Whisk in the dressing ingredients and season with salt and pepper.
- Pour the dressing over the vegetables, add the basil, olives, and pine nuts, and toss lightly.
- Serve warm.

Braised Bok Choy
Serves people: 4
150 cals per serving
Preparation time: 15 minutes
Cooking time: 20 minutes
Instructions:

- 25 ml (1 Fl oz) coconut aminos
- Grated zest and juice of ½ orange
- 30 ml (2 tbsp) rice wine or medium sherry
- 5 ml (1 tsp) grated fresh root ginger
- 1 garlic clove, peeled and crushed
- 1 red chili, deseeded and chopped
- 1 whole-star anise
- 12 small bok choy, trimmed
- 44 ml (3 tbsp) nutritional yeast flakes

Instructions:

- Strip the bok choy and rinse each layer well to eliminate debris. After thoroughly cleaning, chop into bite-size pieces.
- Place all the ingredients, except the bok choy and nutritional yeast, into a wide pan with 60 ml (4 tbsp) water, bring to a boil, cover, and simmer for 15 minutes.
- Add bok choy to the pan and mix with liquid. Cover and simmer for a further 5 minutes until tender. Serve immediately, then toss on nutritional yeast.

Grilled Portobello Mushrooms with Herbs and Garlic
Serves people: 6
185 cals per serving
Preparation time: 10 minutes, plus chilling
Cooking time: 10 minutes
Ingredients:

- 125 g (4 oz) coconut butter
- 2 garlic cloves, peeled and crushed
- 30 ml (2 tbsp) chopped fresh herbs of chives, chervil, parsley, and thyme
- 5 ml (1 tsp) grated lemon zest
- 12 portobello mushrooms, trimmed

- 15 ml (1 tbsp) olive oil
- Celtic salt
- Pepper

Instructions:

- Cream the coconut butter, garlic, herbs, lemon zest, and a pinch of Celtic salt and pepper in a bowl. Cover the mix and refrigerate for at least 30 minutes to allow the flavors to accentuate.
- Brush the mushrooms lightly with oil, arrange gill-side down on the grill pan, and grill under high heat for 5 minutes.
- Cut the flavored butter into small pieces.
- Turn the mushroom gill side up. Place the flavored butter on the gills and grill for 5 minutes until the mushrooms are tender and sizzling. Serve immediately.

Condiments

Guacamole
Serves people: 6
185 cals per serving
Preparation time: 10 minutes
Ingredients:

- 2 large ripe avocados
- 60 ml (4 tbsp) lemon juice
- 4 ripe tomatoes, skinned, deseeded, and chopped
- 2 fresh red chilis, deseeded and finely chopped
- 1 red onion roughly chopped
- 2 garlic cloves, peeled and crushed
- 60 ml (4 tbsp) coriander leaves, roughly chopped
- 15 ml (1 tbsp) extra-virgin olive oil
- Celtic salt

- Pepper

Instructions:

- Halve, stone, and peel the avocados, reserving the stones. Squash and mix the avocado flesh with the lemon juice in a bowl, then stir in the chopped tomatoes, chili, garlic, onions, tomatoes, coriander, and oil. Season generously with salt and pepper.
- Turn into a serving bowl and push the avocado stones into the mixture. Cover and refrigerate until ready to serve.
- Remove the avocado stones from the guacamole and serve.

Tzatziki

Serves people: 8
45 cals per serving
Preparation time: 10 minutes
Ingredients:

- 1 cucumber
- 300 ml (½ pint) coconut yogurt
- 10 ml (2 tsp) extra-virgin olive oil
- 30 ml (2 tbsp) chopped fresh mint
- 1 large garlic clove, peeled and crushed
- Celtic salt
- Pepper

Instructions:

- Halve, deseed, dice the cucumber, and place in a bowl.
- Add the yogurt and oil.
- Stir in the chopped mint and garlic, seasoning with salt and pepper to taste. 4. Cover and chill in the refrigerator until ready to serve.

Harissa

Serves people: 8
114 cals per serving
Preparation time: 30 minutes
Ingredients:

- 7 whole dried Guajillo chiles, deseeded
- 2 large (6 oz) roasted red peppers
- 30 ml (2 tbsp) tomato paste
- 6 cloves of garlic
- 10 ml (2 tsp) coriander
- 10 ml (2 tsp) cumin
- 2.5 ml (½ tsp) cayenne pepper
- 5 ml (1 tsp) smoked paprika
- 1 large lemon, juiced
- 70 ml (4.73 tbsp) extra-virgin olive oil
- Celtic salt
- Pepper

Instructions:

- Soak the dried red Guajillo chili peppers in hot water to rehydrate to turn them into a paste.
- Place the chiles with the roasted red peppers, garlic, tomato paste, spices, salt, pepper, and lemon juice in a food processor and blend.
- Drizzle 60 ml oil as the ingredients mix until they arrive at a chunky paste.
- Remove to a tight lid mason jar. Add a drizzle of 10 ml oil on top to seal it. Chill until ready to serve.
- Refrigerate for up to 3 weeks. 6. Freeze it for later use for up to 1 month.

Snacks

Stuffed Zucchini Boat

Serves people: 8
53 cals per serving
Preparation time: 10 minutes plus standing time
Cooking time: 25 minutes
Instructions:

- 8 zucchinis halved lengthways and scooped
- 2 red bell peppers halved, deseeded, and chopped finely
- 2 large ripe tomatoes, deseeded, chopped finely
- 1 small red onion, finely chopped
- 7 large garlic cloves peeled and crushed
- 125 g (4 oz) Kalamata olives, finely chopped
- 30 ml (2 tbsp) finely chopped oregano
- 2.5 ml (½ tbs) dried Italian seasoning
- 125g (4 oz) (vegan) feta cheese crumbled
- 30 ml (2 tbsp) finely chopped parsley
- Celtic salt
- Pepper

Instructions:

- Preheat the oven to 230ºC (450ºF) mark 8 for 45 - 50 minutes.
- In a medium bowl, combine red bell peppers, tomato, red onion, garlic, olives, oregano, dried Italian seasoning, salt, and pepper to taste.
- Evenly distribute the mixture on each zucchini. Place in a large baking dish and bake for 20 minutes.
- Top with (vegan) feta cheese and broil on high for three more minutes or until the cheese has browned.
- Remove from the oven, sprinkle with parsley, and serve hot or cold.

Smoked Mackerel Pate

Serves people: 6
230 cals per serving
Preparation time: 10 minutes.
Ingredients:

- 300 g (10 oz) hot-smoked mackerel filets
- 50 g (2 oz) coconut butter
- 45 ml (3 tbsp) creamed horseradish
- 30 ml (2 tbsp) single cream
- Pepper

Instructions:

- Skin the mackerel filets and remove small residual bones using a tweezer. Flake the mackerel in a bowl.
- Add the coconut butter, horseradish, and cream.
- Mash with a fork until evenly blended. Season with pepper.
- Spoon the pate into a serving dish and cover with cling film until ready for consumption.

Popcorn

Serves people: 1
249 cals per serving
Preparation time: 5 mins
Ingredients:

- 45 ml (3 tbsp) avocado oil
- 41.6 g (1.47 oz) high-quality popcorn kernels
- 0.68 g (0.02 oz) Celtic salt
- 10 ml (2 tsp) Paprika (optional)

Instructions:

- Heat the oil on high heat in a 4-quart saucepan.

- Place two popcorn kernels into the oil and cover the pan.
- After the kernels pop, add the rest of the popcorn kernels in an even layer and shake to mix with oil. Cover tightly with a lid.
- Remove entirely from heat when the popping relaxes to a few seconds between pops.
- Once the popping stops, sprinkle Celtic salt to taste.
- Remove the popcorn immediately into a wide bowl. Add paprika (optional).
- Alternatively, air pop the corn kernels, then add salt and (or) paprika.

Chocolate Seamoss Nut Bliss

Serves people: 16
250 cals per serving
Preparation time: 20 minutes
Ingredients:

- 476 g (16.80 oz) dates
- 227 g (8 oz) sea moss gel
- 160 g (5.6 oz) hemp seeds
- 133 g (4.7 oz) Brazil nuts
- 96 g (3.39 oz) desiccated coconut
- 60 ml (4 tbsp) cacao powder
- 30 ml (2 tbsp) ground ginger

Instructions:

- Combine all ingredients except cacao powder in a food processor and blend until glutinous.
- Scoop 1 tablespoon and roll into a ball.
- Coat the ball with cacao powder.
- Place in an airtight container.
- Repeat steps 2 - 4 until completed.

- Place the container in the refrigerator until hardened and ready to eat.
- Refrigerate for up to one week!

Desserts

Sea Moss Gel base for desserts, teas, cooking and eating raw
30 ml (2 tbsp) = 15 cals per person per day.
Ingredients:

- 100 g (3.5 oz) Irish Moss
- 7 cups warm water for soaking the sea moss

Instructions:

- Cleanse the sea moss: Place the sea moss in a colander. Use vigorous hand movements to thoroughly wash debris and excess sea salt from the sea moss. Rinse twice.
- In a large bowl, place the sea moss in 7 cups of room temperature water and leave to soak for 24 hours. The sea moss will expand in size.
- Drain soaking water off the sea moss.
- Prepare the gel: Place the sea moss into a blender, gradually add purified, filtered, or spring water, and puree into a gel. Ensure the puree is completely smooth without sea moss granules, dissolved into a gelatinous texture.
- Transfer the gel into a mason jar and refrigerate it for everyday use. The gel lasts one month in the refrigerator and six months frozen.

Chia Moss Mousse
Serves people: 2
197 cals per serving
Preparation time: 5 minutes
Ingredients:

- 237 ml (8.5 oz) almond milk
- 30 ml (2 tbsp) sea moss gel
- 30 ml (2 tbsp) chia seeds
- 5 ml (1 tsp) ground nutmeg
- 5 ml (1 tsp) ground cinnamon
- 5 ml (1 tsp) vanilla extract

Instructions:

- In a blender, combine all the ingredients and process until smooth. Remove to a mason jar and refrigerate or indulge in a serving glass.

Sea Moss Berry Smoothie
Serves people: 4
166 cals per serving
Preparation time: 5 minutes
Ingredients:

- 1 L (35 oz) almond milk
- 237 ml (5.8 oz) mixed frozen berries of strawberries, blueberries, blackberries, and raspberries
- 148 ml (5 oz) coconut yogurt
- 30 ml (2 tbsp) sea moss gel
- 30 ml (2 tbsp) chia seeds
- 5 ml (1 tsp) nutmeg
- 5 ml (1 tsp) ground cinnamon
- 5 ml (1 tsp) vanilla extract

Instructions:

- In a blender, combine all the ingredients and process until smooth.
- Add ice cubes (optional).
- Remove to a serving glass and indulge.

Pinabananice

Serves people: 3
440 cals per serving
Preparation time: 5 hours plus standing time
Ingredients:

- 1065 ml (4.5 cups) 1 large pineapple, peeled, cubed, and frozen
- 2 large ripe bananas, sliced and frozen
- 300 ml (10.9 oz) almond milk
- 10 ml (2 tsp) vanilla extract
- 5 ml (1 tsp) spirulina
- 5 ml (1 tsp) cinnamon
- 2.5 ml (½ tsp) organic green stevia leaves powder

Instructions:

- In a blender, combine all the ingredients and process until smooth.
- Pour the contents into a freezer container and refreeze for 4 hours.
- Remove from the freezer, leave to soften, and break into chunks. Return to the blender and churn.
- Pour the blend back into the freezer container and freeze for 1 hour before serving.
- To serve: If the blend is too hard to scoop, allow it to defrost at room temperature for 2 minutes until easy to scoop.

Beverages

Spice Detox Infusion

Serves people: 4
64 cals per serving
Preparation: 15 minutes plus standing time

Ingredients:

- 1.5 L (50.72 Fl oz) water
- 10 large barks of cinnamon sticks
- 60 ml (4 tbsp) apple cider vinegar
- Juice of 4 lemons
- 30 ml (2 tbsp) sea moss gel
- 60 ml (4 tbsp) ground ginger
- 30 ml (2 tbsp) ground cinnamon
- 5 ml (1 tsp) dash of cayenne pepper
- 5 ml (1 tsp) vanilla extract

Instructions:

- Place cinnamon sticks in a pot of water and bring to a boil. Infuse on a low boil for another 10 minutes.
- Remove from heat and add sea moss gel, ginger, cinnamon, and cayenne pepper.
- Let cool, and add apple cider vinegar and lemon juice.
- Serve warm or cold.
- Store in the refrigerator with cinnamon sticks; the beverage will get sweeter as if sweetened with sugar.

Smooth Green Blend

Serves people: 4
142 cals per serving
Preparation time: 15 minutes
Ingredients:

- 1 cup (8 Fl oz) avocado flesh
- 1 cup (8 Fl oz) fresh chopped celery
- 1 cup (8 Fl oz) fresh spinach
- 1 cup (8 Fl oz) chopped fresh kale
- 5 ml (1 tsp) spirulina
- 1 cup (8Fl oz) cucumber, chopped

- 1 L (33.81 Fl oz) coconut water or filtered water
- 2.5 ml (½ tsp) organic green stevia leaves powder (optional for sweet taste)

Instructions:

- In a blender, combine all the ingredients and process until smooth.
- Salivate and consume slowly.

Dairy-Free Cini Chocolate

Serves people: 1
64 cals per serving
Preparation time: 15 minutes plus standing time
Ingredients:

- 950 ml (32 Fl oz) water
- 7 large cinnamon sticks
- 30 ml (2 tbsp) ground cinnamon
- 30 ml (2 tbsp) lemon juice
- 15 ml (1 tbsp) raw unpasteurized natural honey

Instructions:

- Place water in a pot and add cinnamon sticks. Bring to a boil.
- Place on low heat and add cinnamon powder. Boil for 10 minutes.
- Remove from heat.
- Allow to cool, then add lemon juice and raw honey. Adding honey after the drink is cool is healthiest. Enjoy at warm to room temperature or cold.

Cinnamon Fat Burner

Serves people: 4

130 cals per serving
Preparation time: 15 minutes plus standing time
Ingredients:

- 4 green apples
- 3 lemons
- 2 large cinnamon sticks
- 1-litre water

Instructions:

- Halve, deseed, and dice apples.
- Wash and scrub the skin of the lemon. Halve, deseed, and dice the lemons.
- Place apples and lemons in a pot. Top with water and bring to a boil. Boil for a further 10 minutes on low heat.
- Place cinnamon sticks in a glass or stainless-steel drinks container. Sieve the hot apple-lemon water into the container and close the lid to brew for at least 30 mins. The longer the brew, the sweeter the beverage.
- Serve warm or cold.

Ginger Honey Lemonade

Serves people: 1
53 cals per serving
Preparation time: 5 minutes.
Ingredients:

- 45 ml (3 tbsp) lemon juice
- 30 ml (2 tbsp) juice of ginger
- 15 ml (1 tbsp) honey
- 250 ml (8.8 Fl oz) water

Instructions:

- Combine the juice of freshly squeezed lemons, freshly juiced ginger root, and honey in a glass of water.
- Stir well and consume it at room temperature or cold.

Added Bonus: Finger-lickin' Indian Recipes

Breakfast

With IF, the most important meal is the first one you eat after long fasting hours, no matter what time of day you choose. It is effortless to lose track and over-eat at this stage. But fret not. I have your back. Here are two healthy and quick recipes that work best with an IF regime.

FRUITS + RAVA (Semolina) Idli + Tomato/Coriander Chutney

Serves people: 2
301 cals per serving
Preparation time: 10 mins
Cooking time: 15 mins
Ingredients:

- 1 cup rava/semolina/suji (coarse)
- 15 ml (3 tsp) oil
- 5 ml (1 tsp) mustard seeds
- 5 ml (1 tsp) chana dal
- 5 cashews
- 2.5 ml (½ tsp) cumin seeds
- A pinch of asafoetida
- A few curry leaves (5-7)
- 1 chili (finely chopped)
- 1-inch ginger (finely chopped)
- 10 ml (2 tbsp) carrot (grated)
- 10 ml (2 tbsp) coriander (finely chopped)

- 1 ml (¼ tsp) turmeric
- 177 ml (¾ cup) curd yogurt (whisked)
- 0.08 oz (½ tsp) salt
- 2.5 ml (½) cup water
- 1 ml (¼) tsp eno/fruit salt

Instructions:

- Heat oil in a pan, then add mustard, cumin, and chana dal.
- Next, add asafoetida and a few curry leaves.
- Add the chili and ginger and sauté for 1-2 minutes.
- Add the chopped carrots and continue stirring.
- Add the turmeric and mix well.
- Lower the flame and add the rava. Take time and roast it thoroughly until there is an aroma.
- Transfer the rava to the bowl and allow cooling.
- Add the curd, coriander, salt, and water to a smooth batter.
- Rest the mixture for 15 minutes and let the rava soak in the water.
- Add Eno/fruit salt to the combination so that it fluffs up easily.
- Steam the batter in the idli maker for 13 minutes.
- Enjoy with fresh fruits and tomato/coriander chutney!

Oats + **M**oong **Dal Chilla**

Serves people: 1
704 cals per serving
Preparation time: 10 minutes
Cooking time: 25minutes
Ingredients:

- 4 oz (½ cup) moong dal
- 4 oz (½ cup) powdered oats

- 0.04 oz (¼ tsp) of cumin
- 1-inch grated ginger (as per taste)
- 120 ml (½ cup) water (to soak the dal overnight)
- 7 ml (½ tbsp) of ghee or oil
- 15 g (¼ cup) carrots
- 1 sprig (20 g) coriander, roughly chopped for garnish
- 1 fresh red chili (chopped) - optional
- Celtic salt to taste

Instructions:

- Add the moong dal to a bowl and rinse water until the water runs clear.
- Soak the moong dal in water for 15-20 minutes so they swell up.
- Chop the veggies in the meanwhile.
- After 20 minutes, add the soaked dal, coriander, and chilies to the blender.
- Blend to form a smooth paste.
- Add the powdered oats, chopped carrots, and salt to taste to the paste.
- Heat ghee/oil in a pan and spread the paste in a round shape.
- Fry lightly on both sides until there is some browning.
- Eat it hot and fresh with tomato chutney or yogurt dip for the perfect balance.

Lunch

Balancing your lunch can be tricky during the IF diet. Your lunch needs to be light, nutritious, and properly portioned. The following two recipes work best for this purpose.

Brown Rice + Rajma + Curd

Serves people: 2
38 cals per serving
Preparation time: 20 mins
Cooking time: 20 mins
Ingredients:

- 10 ml (2 tsp) oil or ghee
- 8 oz (1 cup) overnight-soaked kidney beans (rajma)
- 8 oz (1 cup) brown rice
- 4 oz (½ cup) chopped onion
- 1 tomato chopped
- 1 inch ginger chopped
- 4-5 cloves of garlic chopped
- 1 bay leaf
- 1 ml (¼ tsp) turmeric powder
- 5 ml (½ tsp) ground cumin
- 5 ml (½ tsp) paprika
- 1 ml (¼ tsp) black pepper
- 15 ml (1 tsp) garam masala
- 15 ml (1 tsp) lemon juice
- 120 ml (½ cup) curd

Instructions:

- In a pot or a pressure cooker, heat oil or ghee.
- Add the bay leaf when the oil/ghee starts simmering.
- Add the chopped onions and sauté it until brown.
- Add the ginger and garlic and caramelize until the aroma is detectable.
- Add in all the ground spices and keep stirring.
- Add warm water and then the chopped tomatoes.
- Cover the pot and cook on low heat for 15 minutes.
- Meanwhile, wash the brown rice and cook it for 15 minutes.
- Finally, add some lemon juice before serving.

- Fill your plate with one-third rice, half with rajma, and the rest with curd, and enjoy!

Vegetable Salad + Rice + Tofu Curry
Serves people: 2
70 cals per serving
Preparation time: 3 minutes
Cooking time: 17 minutes
Ingredients:

- 200g firm tofu
- 8 oz (1 cup) rice
- 1 onion diced
- 2 bell peppers diced
- 1 tomato chopped
- 15 ml (1 tbsp) olive oil
- 2.5 ml (½ tsp) turmeric
- 2 cloves of garlic, chopped
- 30 ml (2 tbsp) of corn-starch
- 5 ml (1 tsp) pepper
- 5 ml (1 tsp) ground cumin
- 5 ml (1 tsp) garam masala
- Salt and sugar to taste
- 2 cups of water
- 250 g lettuce (blanched)
- 1 cucumber (cut in rounds)
- 250 g spinach (blanched)

Instructions:

- Wash and cook the measured rice while the tofu cooks.
- Drain the water away from the tofu and cut it into cubes.
- Add cornstarch, salt, and pepper; coat the tofu cubes in a bowl.

- Heat one tablespoon of oil in a pan and fry the coated tofu.
- Once golden brown, set the tofu aside.
- Add the onions to the same pan and sauté them with bell peppers and tomatoes.
- Add the garlic and mix well.
- Add the tofu once the veggies are half-cooked.
- Add the grounded spices and stir well.
- Add some water and chopped tomatoes and cover the pan.
- Cook on low heat for 12 minutes.
- Blanch the lettuce and spinach for 3-5 minutes.
- Fill your plate with ⅓ rice, ½ tofu curry, and the rest with salad. Enjoy this well-balanced meal in under 20 minutes of cooking.

Dinner

Chicken Stew + Roti/Rice + Salad

Serves people: 2
669 cals per serving
Preparation time: 15 minutes
Cooking time: 30 minutes
Ingredients:

- Chicken pieces (2-5) with bone
- 8 oz (1 cup) rice
- Lettuce/ salad leaves
- Fresh cucumber (in discs)
- 1 carrot, diced
- 4 potatoes, halved
- 2 onions, diced
- 1 tomato, chopped
- 1 large bell pepper, chopped
- 1-inch ginger finely chopped
- 4 cloves of garlic, chopped

- 30 ml (2 tbsp) oil
- Spring onions, optional
- Salt and pepper to taste

Instructions:

- Heat oil/ butter in a pan and fry the chicken lightly until it becomes yellowish-brown; set aside.
- In the same pan, add the veggies and stir until they become translucent.
- Add the ginger and garlic and keep stirring.
- Add salt and pepper.
- Re-add the chicken pieces and stir well with the veggies.
- Add a 1/2 cup of water and cover the pan; cook for 20-25 minutes to ensure thorough cooking of the chicken.
- Meanwhile, wash and cook the rice for 15 minutes. If opting for roti, you can prepare it while the chicken cooks. Roti's instructions are below.
- Once done, garnish with spring onions.
- Fill your plate with the chicken stew, followed by ⅓ of the plate with rice or two rotis. Load up on the sliced lettuce and cucumbers to make it a wholesome meal!

Broccoli Salad + Roti+ Mix Vegetable Curry
Serves people: 2
960 cals per serving
Preparation time: 10 minutes
Cooking time: 25 minutes
Ingredients:

- Half a cauliflower, cut in florets
- Half a broccoli, cut in florets
- 4 potatoes, chopped
- 200 g French beans, chopped
- 2 carrots, chopped

- 2 onions, diced
- 1 tomato, chopped
- 1 tablespoon cumin seeds
- 2 tablespoons oil
- 3 cloves garlic, chopped
- 1-inch of ginger, chopped

Dough prepared for 2-4 rotis

- 0.25 oz (½ tbsp) turmeric
- 0.25 oz (½ tbsp) paprika powder
- 24 oz (3 cups) whole wheat flour
- Celtic salt to taste

Instructions:

- Heat oil in a pan.
- Splatter cumin seeds in the hot oil to brown.
- Then, add cauliflower, beans, carrots, and onions sequentially.
- Add salt and sauté until all the veggies change color.
- Add the ginger and garlic.
- Add the turmeric and paprika powder and mix everything well.
- Add the tomatoes.
- Add 1/2 cup of water and cover the pan for 15 minutes.
- In another pan, blanch the broccoli with some salt for 7 minutes.
- Take out the broccoli and garnish with salt and pepper.
- Prepare the roti while the veggies are cooking.
- After 15 minutes, keep stir-frying the veggies to gain the proper consistency.
- Fill your plate with ½ mixed veggies, ¼ with roti, and ¼ with broccoli salad for the perfect nutritious meal.

To make roti:

- Knead the roti dough by mixing a tsp of salt and flour. Ensure that the consistency of the dough is such that you can roll a flattened roti out of it.
- Keep the griddle or iron skillet on medium heat.
- Meanwhile, make a small ball out of the dough and roll it with the help of a rolling pin.
- Place the flattened dough on the griddle and let it cook evenly from both sides.
- Roti will begin to puff. Use a clean cloth to gently press the roti so it gets cooked evenly.
- Place the cooked roti on a dish and apply butter/ghee.

ACCOUNTABILITY

"The things that are easy to do are also easy *not* to do. That's the difference between success and failure, between daydreams and ambitions."

— JIM ROHN

NOTES

Chapter 1: Intermittent Fasting: Your Bridge to Your Ideal Body

Ajmera, R. (2023, March 13). 8 Health benefits of fasting, backed by science. *Healthline.* https://www.healthline.com/nutrition/fasting-benefits.

Barnosky, A. R., Hoddy, K. K., Unterman, T. G., & Varady, K. A. (2014, June 12). Intermittent fasting vs daily calorie restriction for type 2 diabetes prevention: A review of human findings. *Translational Research, 164*(4), 302–311. https://doi.org/10.1016/j.trsl.2014.05.013.

BSc, K. G. (2019, July 22). 11 Myths about fasting and meal frequency. *Healthline.* https://www.healthline.com/nutrition/11-myths-fasting-and-meal-frequency#TOC_TITLE_HDR_13.

Eenfeldt, A. (2020, August 29). How to maximize fat burning. *Diet Doctor.* https://www.dietdoctor.com/how-to-maximize-fat-burning.

Eenfeldt, A. (2022, November 4). Learn intermittent fasting - Video course. *Diet Doctor.* https://www.dietdoctor.com/learn-intermittent-fasting-new-video-course.

Lapine, P. (2017, May 16). How to eat better (without breaking the bank). *Better by Today.* https://www.nbcnews.com/better/diet-fitness/11-ways-eat-better-cheaper-summer-n759571.

Lean, M. E., Leslie, W. S., Barnes, A. C., Brosnahan, N., Thom, G., McCombie, L., Peters, C., Zhyzhneuskaya, S., Al-Mrabeh, A., Hollingsworth, K. G., Rodrigues, A. M., Rehackova, L., Adamson, A. J., Sniehotta, F. F., Mathers, J. C., Ross, H. M., McIlvenna, Y., Stefanetti, R., Trenell, M., & Welsh, P. (2018, February 10). Primary care-led weight management for remission of type 2 diabetes (DiRECT): An open label, cluster-randomised trial. *The Lancet, 391*(10120), 541–551. https://doi.org/10.1016/s0140-6736(17)33102-1

Link, R. (2023, March 9). Intermittent fasting: How to do it for weight loss. *Dr. Axe.* https://draxe.com/nutrition/intermittent-fasting-benefits.

Nazish, N. (2021, June 30). 10 Intermittent fasting myths you should stop believing. *Forbes.* https://www.forbes.com/sites/nomanazish/2021/06/30/10-intermittent-fasting-myths-you-should-stop-believing/?sh=27163997335b.

Pytlewicz, M. (2020, June 16). Intermittent fasting, autophagy and physical changes in the body. *Delos Therapy.* https://delostherapy.com/intermittent-fasting-autophagy-and-physical-changes-in-the-body/?sfw=pass1659424500.

The Nobel Prize in Physiology or Medicine 2016. (2016, October 3). Press release. *The Nobel Prize.* https://www.nobelprize.org/prizes/medicine/2016/press-release.

Chapter 2: Hormone Harmonization & Resurrecting The 12 Systems

Altshuler, M. (2009, May 4). The bad news is time flies; The good news is you're the pilot. *Northern Lakes Community Mental Health Authority*. https://www.northernlakescmh.org/inspirational-poems-and-prose/inspirational-quotes/the-bad-news-is-time-flies-the-good-news-is-youre-the-pilot-michael-altshuler.

Axe, J. (2022, September 15). 6 Steps for how to balance hormones naturally. *Dr. Axe*. https://draxe.com/health/how-to-balance-hormones-naturally.

Brittain, K. (2020, October 26). Fasting and the immune system: What you need to know. *Well Wisdom*. https://www.wellwisdom.com/fasting-and-the-immune-system-what-you-need-to-know.

Faris, S. (2017, February 14). Late-onset menopause: What is causing your delay? *Healthline*. https://www.healthline.com/health/menopause/late-onset#Pregnancy-and-late-onset-menopause.

Fung, J. MD. (2022, March 23). My single best weight loss tip. *Diet Doctor*. https://www.dietdoctor.com/my-single-best-weight-loss-tip.

Group, N. A.-T. I. (2020, October 13). Can we reset the Grim Reaper™ clock? *Neurological Associates The Interventional Group | Santa Monica & Los Angeles*. https://www.neurologysantamonica.com/can-we-reset-the-grim-reaper-clock.

Gudden, J., Arias Vasquez, A., & Bloemendaal, M. (2021, September 10). The effects of intermittent fasting on brain and cognitive function. *Nutrients, 13*(9), 3166. https://doi.org/10.3390/nu13093166.

Johnson, J. (n.d.). How to boost your leptin levels. *Webber Naturals Canada*. https://www.webbernaturals.com/en-ca/learn/how-to-boost-your-leptin-levels.

Kim, B. H., Joo, Y., Kim, M.-S., Choe, H. K., Tong, Q., & Kwon, O. (2021, August 27). Effects of intermittent fasting on the circulating levels and circadian rhythms of hormones. *Endocrinology and Metabolism, 36*(4), 745–756. https://doi.org/10.3803/enm.2021.405.

Malinowski, B., Zalewska, K., Węsierska, A., Sokołowska, M. M., Socha, M., Liczner, G., Pawlak-Osińska, K., & Wiciński, M. (2019, March 20). Intermittent fasting in cardiovascular disorders—An overview. *Nutrients, 11*(3), 673. https://doi.org/10.3390/nu11030673.

Mba, A. L. B. (2022, January 31). 10 natural ways to balance your hormones. *Healthline*. https://www.healthline.com/nutrition/balance-hormones.

National Institute on Aging. (2020). Understanding the dynamics of the aging process. *National Institute on Aging*. https://www.nia.nih.gov/about/aging-strategic-directions-research/understanding-dynamics-aging.

National Institute of Aging. (2021). What Is Menopause? *National Institute on Aging*. https://www.nia.nih.gov/health/what-menopause#transition.

NHS. (2022, May 17). Overview - Menopause. *NHS*. https://www.nhs.uk/conditions/menopause.

NT Contributor. (2017, July 31). Anatomy and physiology of ageing 7: The endocrine system. *Nursing Times.* https://www.nursingtimes.net/roles/older-people-nurses-roles/anatomy-and-physiology-of-ageing-7-the-endocrine-system-31-07-2017.

Phillips, M. C. (2019, October 17). Fasting as a therapy in neurological disease. *Nutrients, 11*(10), 2501. https://doi.org/10.3390/nu11102501.

Prisco, S. Z., Eklund, M., Moutsoglou, D. M., Prisco, A. R., Khoruts, A., Weir, E. K., Thenappan, T., & Prins, K. W. (2021, November 16). Intermittent fasting enhances right ventricular function in preclinical pulmonary arterial hypertension. *Journal of the American Heart Association, 10*(22). https://doi.org/10.1161/jaha.121.022722.

Ruggeri, C. (2017, June 21). The insulin resistance diet protocol. *Dr. Axe.* https://draxe.com/health/insulin-resistance-diet.

WebMD Editorial Contributors. (2021, March 18). What to know about heavy bleeding after 50. *WebMD.* https://www.webmd.com/healthy-aging/heavy-bleeding-after-50#:~:text=Bleeding%20can%20occur%20in%20women,most%20common%20among%20postmenopausal%20women.

Wu, S. (2014, June 5). Fasting triggers stem cell regeneration of damaged, old immune system. *USC News.* http://news.usc.edu/63669/fasting-triggers-stem-cell-regeneration-of-damaged-old-immune-system.

Chapter 3: Breaking Through The Barriers

Abbasi, B., Kimiagar, M., Sadeghniiat, K., Shirazi, M. M., Hedayati, M., & Rashidkhani, B. (2012, December). The effect of magnesium supplementation on primary insomnia in elderly: A double-blind placebo-controlled clinical trial. *Journal of Research in Medical Sciences: The Official Journal of Isfahan University of Medical Sciences, 17*(12), 1161-1169. https://www.ncbi.nlm.nih.gov/pmc/articles/PMC3703169.

Breus, D. M. (2022, December 13). Aging and sleep. *The Sleep Doctor.* https://thesleepdoctor.com/aging.

Breus, D. M. (2022, September 9). How to fall asleep fast. *The Sleep Doctor.* https://thesleepdoctor.com/sleep-hygiene/how-to-fall-asleep-fast.

Collins, D. (2021, July 12). The power of music to reduce stress. *Psych Central.* https://psychcentral.com/stress/the-power-of-music-to-reduce-stress#:~:text=Music%20to%20reduce%20anxiety&text=In%20one%20study%20of%20over,levels%20also%20helps%20tackle%20anxiety.

Hirotsu, C., Tufik, S., & Andersen, M. L. (2015, November). Interactions between sleep, stress, and metabolism: From physiological to pathological conditions. *Sleep Science, 8*(3), 143-152. https://doi.org/10.1016/j.slsci.2015.09.002.

How to overcome food addiction: Eating for strength | *BetterHelp.* (n.d.). https://www.betterhelp.com/advice/eating-disorders/how-to-overcome-food-addiction-eating-for-strength.

Jennings, K.-A. (2022, January 20). 15 simple ways to relieve stress. *Healthline.* https://www.healthline.com/nutrition/16-ways-relieve-stress-anxiety#The-bottom-line.

Levy, J. (2015, August 9). Mindful eating: Maintain a healthy weight & appetite. *Dr. Axe*. Draxe.com. https://draxe.com/health/mindful-eating.

Mayo Clinic Staff. (2022, November 22). Forgiveness: Letting go of grudges and bitterness. *Mayo Clinic*. https://www.mayoclinic.org/healthy-lifestyle/adult-health/in-depth/forgiveness/art-20047692.

Paul, R. (2015, March 23). Proverb for the day 23:19-21 - Too much meat, too much wine. . .Not enough listening! *Helping up Mission*. https://helpingupmission.org/2015/03/proverb-for-the-day-2319-21-too-much-meat-too-much-wine-not-enough-listening.

Satrazemis, E. (2021, March 23). What is body composition? And 5 ways to measure body fat. *Trifecta*. https://www.trifectanutrition.com/blog/what-is-body-composition-and-how-to-measure-it.

Scott, E., PhD. (2022, October 19). 18 effective stress relief strategies. *Verywell Mind*. https://www.verywellmind.com/tips-to-reduce-stress-3145195.

University of Colorado. (2014, December 16). 25 quick ways to reduce stress. *Colorado Law*. https://www.colorado.edu/law/25-quick-ways-reduce-stress.

Weiner, Z. (2017, March 22). 7 tips for eliminating toxic people from your life. *Mental Floss*. https://www.mentalfloss.com/article/93521/7-tips-eliminating-toxic-people-your-life.

Wiesel, E. (2006). *Night*. Translated by M. Wiesel. New York, NY: Hill & Wang.

Chapter 4 Conscious Intermittent Fasting Formula: When - Step 1

Aleknavičius, K. (2023, April 7). Dr. Jason Fung's fasting methods. *DoFasting*. https://dofasting.com/blog/jason-fung-fasting.

Baum, I. (2022, February 4). What happens to your body when you don't drink enough water. *EatingWell*. https://www.eatingwell.com/article/292133/10-dangerous-side-effects-of-not-drinking-enough-water.

Bueno, S. (2018, April 20). How proper hydration affects bone health. *Watauga Orthopaedics*. https://www.wataugaortho.com/2018/04/20/how-proper-hydration-affects-bone-health.

Franklin, J. (n.d.). Nine reasons for fasting. *Jentezen Franklin*. https://jfm-website.s3.amazonaws.com/fasting/article/Nine-Reasons.pdf.

Jamshed, H., Beyl, R. A., Della Manna, D. L., Yang, E. S., Ravussin, E., & Peterson, C. M. (2019, May 30). Early time-restricted feeding improves 24-hour glucose levels and affects markers of the circadian clock, aging, and autophagy in humans. *Nutrients, 11*(6), 1234. https://doi.org/10.3390/nu11061234.

Jones, R., Pabla, P., Mallinson, J., Nixon, A., Taylor, T., Bennett, A., & Tsintzas, K. (2020, October). Two weeks of early time-restricted feeding (eTRF) improves skeletal muscle insulin and anabolic sensitivity in healthy men. *The American Journal of Clinical Nutrition, 112*(4), 1015-1028. https://doi.org/10.1093/ajcn/nqaa192.

Kiltz, R. (2022, January 3). Circadian rhythm fasting: Everything you need to know.

Doctor Kiltz. https://www.doctorkiltz.com/circadian-rhythm-fasting/#:~:text=Both%20circadian%20rhythm%20fasting%20and,as%20the%2016%3A8%20method.

- Morin, K. (2022, January 28). 5 intermittent fasting methods: Which one is right for you? *Life by Daily Burn.* https://dailyburn.com/life/health/intermittent-fasting-methods.
- Mph, C. S. (2022, March 3). What is metabolic flexibility and how can you achieve it? *Bulletproof.* https://www.bulletproof.com/diet/weight-loss/metabolic-flexibility.
- Ravussin, E., Beyl, R. A., Poggiogalle, E., Hsia, D. S., & Peterson, C. M. (2019, July 24). Early time-restricted feeding reduces appetite and increases fat oxidation but does not affect energy expenditure in humans. *Obesity, 27*(8), 1244–1254. https://doi.org/10.1002/oby.22518.
- RDN, M. K., MS. (2021, November 8). Circadian rhythm fasting: Eating to align with your internal clock. *InsideTracker.* https://blog.insidetracker.com/circadian-rhythm-fasting.
- Reck, T. (2022, December 19). Intermittent fasting plans for beginners. *Simple.* https://simple.life/blog/intermittent-fasting-plans.
- Snyder, C., & Gunners, K. (2022, February 23). Pros and cons of 5 intermittent fasting methods. *Healthline.* https://www.healthline.com/nutrition/6-ways-to-do-intermittent-fasting#bottom-line.
- Sutton, E. F., Beyl, R., Early, K. S., Cefalu, W. T., Ravussin, E., & Peterson, C. M. (2018, June 5). Early time-restricted feeding improves insulin sensitivity, blood pressure, and oxidative stress even without weight loss in men with prediabetes. *Cell Metabolism, 27*(6), 1212-1221.e3. https://doi.org/10.1016/j.cmet.2018.04.010.
- Trumpfeller, G. (2020, May 15). 7 treacherous intermittent fasting mistakes (and how to avoid them). *Simple.* https://simple.life/blog/intermittent-fasting-mistakes.
- Young, C. (2017, October 25). How to fast (without losing your mind or muscles). *Ample.* https://www.amplemeal.com/blogs/home/how-to-fast.

Chapter 5: Conscious Feasting: What to Eat - Step 2

- Axe, J. (2023, April 10). Sea salt vs. table salt: Benefits, types, uses, side effects & more. *Dr. Axe.* https://draxe.com/nutrition/sea-salt.
- Axe, J. (2023, February 21). Keto diet for beginners: The ultimate guide to keto. *Dr. Axe.* https://draxe.com/nutrition/guide-to-keto-diet-for-beginners.
- Eckelkamp, S. (2022, June 7). Intermittent fasting? Here's exactly what to eat at the end of your fast. *Mbghealth.* https://www.mindbodygreen.com/articles/intermittent-fasting-heres-right-way-to-break-your-fast.
- Hullett, A. (2021, March 25). Should you be using sea moss for weight loss? *Greatist.* https://greatist.com/live/sea-moss-for-weight-loss#how-to-use.
- Levy, J. (2023, January 4). Top 11 leafy greens (& their health benefits). *Dr. Axe.* https://draxe.com/nutrition/leafy-greens.

Link, R. (2023, February 1). Cruciferous vegetables: Cancer killer or thyroid killer? Benefits, recipes, side effects. *Dr. Axe*. https://draxe.com/nutrition/cruciferous-vegetables.

McAuliffe, L. (2021, December 31). The Mediterranean keto diet: What is it and what to eat? *Doctor Kiltz*. https://www.doctorkiltz.com/mediterranean-keto-diet.

National Cancer Institute. (2010). Cruciferous vegetables and cancer prevention. *National Cancer Institute*. https://www.cancer.gov/about-cancer/causes-prevention/risk/diet/cruciferous-vegetables-fact-sheet.

Pitchford, P. (2009). *Healing with whole foods: Asian traditions and modern nutrition (3rd ed.)*. Berkeley, Calif: North Atlantic Books.

Publishing H. H. (2021, February 15). Low fat, low carb, or Mediterranean: Which diet is right for you? *Harvard Health*. https://www.health.harvard.edu/staying-healthy/low-fat-low-carb-or-mediterranean-which-diet-is-right-for-you.

Schilling, R. (2022, February 13). How healthy are carbohydrates? *Medical Articles by Dr. Ray*. https://www.askdrray.com/tag/mediterranean-diet.

Sweeney, E. (2022, December 14). 110 foods you can eat on the Mediterranean diet—from hummus to beets to ... Octopus? *Parade: Entertainment, Recipes, Health, Life, Holidays*. https://parade.com/983137/ericasweeney/mediterranean-diet-food-list.

Younkin, L. (2019, December 19). Mediterranean diet for beginners: Everything you need to get started. *EatingWell*. https://www.eatingwell.com/article/291120/mediterranean-diet-for-beginners-everything-you-need-to-get-started.

Chapter 6: Dance to the Right Tune: Enough is Enough

Ali R, Hashmi MF, Patel C. (2023, February 19). Milk-Alkali syndrome. *StatPearls Publishing. PubMed*. https://pubmed.ncbi.nlm.nih.gov/32491432.

Ames, B. N. (n.d.) The "Triage theory": Micronutrient deficiencies cause insidious damage that accelerates age-associated chronic disease. *Bruce N. Ames*. http://www.bruceames.org/Triage.pdf.

Cordeiro, B. (2014, March). 7 exercise myths debunked. *MD Anderson Cancer Center*. https://www.mdanderson.org/publications/focused-on-health/exercise-myths.h12-1589046.html.

Cranenburg, E. C. M., Vermeer, C., Koos, R., Boumans, M., Hacking, T. M., Bouwman, F. G., Kwaijtaal, M., Brandenburg, V., Ketteler, M., & Schurgers, L. J. (2008, August). The circulating inactive form of matrix Gla protein (ucMGP) as a biomarker for cardiovascular calcification. *Journal of Vascular Research, 45*(5), 427-436. https://doi.org/10.1159/000124863.

Geleijnse, J. M., Vermeer, C., Grobbee, D. E., Schurgers, L. J., Knapen, M. H., van der Meer, I. M., Hofman, A., & Witteman, J. C. (2004, November). Dietary intake of menaquinone is associated with a reduced risk of coronary heart disease: The Rotterdam study. *The Journal of Nutrition, 134*(11), 3100-3105. https://doi.org/10.1093/jn/134.11.3100.

Gennev. (n.d.). Menopause and weight or resistance training. *Integrated care for menopause.* https://www.gennev.com/education/weight-resistance-training-menopause.

Manna, P., & Kalita, J. (2016, July). Beneficial role of vitamin K supplementation on insulin sensitivity, glucose metabolism, and the reduced risk of type 2 diabetes: A review. *Nutrition, 32*(7-8), 732-739. https://doi.org/10.1016/j.nut.2016.01.011.

Mishra, N., & Mishra, V. N. (2011, July 1). Exercise beyond menopause: Dos and don'ts. *Journal of Mid-Life Health, 2*(2), 51-56. https://doi.org/10.4103/0976-7800.92524.

NHS. (2017, October 23). Vitamin K. *NHS.* https://www.nhs.uk/conditions/vitamins-and-minerals/vitamin-k.

Osteocalcin ELISA kit: Gla-type osteocalcin (Gla-OC) EIA Kit. (n.d.). *Takara.* https://www.takarabio.com/products/antibodies-and-elisa/primary-antibodies-and-elisas-by-research-area/bone-research/osteocalcin-carboxylated-gla-oc.

Pitchford, P. (2009). *Healing with whole foods: Asian traditions and modern nutrition (3rd ed.).* Berkeley, Calif: North Atlantic Books.

Recombinant Human Uncarboxylated Osteocalcin (ELISA Std.). (2019, November 27). *BioLegend.* https://www.biolegend.com/en-us/products/recombinant-human-uncarboxylated-osteocalcin-elisa-std-18703?pdf=true&displayInline=true&leftRightMargin=15&topBottomMargin=15&filename=Recombinant%20Human%20Uncarboxylated%20Osteocalcin%20(ELISA%20Std.).pdf&v=20230114013553.

Snegarov, Y. S. (2019, April 15). GLA proteins – The warning sign for the blood vessels. *Journal of IMAB.* https://journal-imab-bg.org/issues-2019/issue2/JofIMAB-2019-25-2p2491-2497.pdf.

Sultana, H., Watanabe, K., Rana, M. M., Takashima, R., Ohashi, A., Komai, M., & Shirakawa, H. (2018, July 27). Effects of vitamin K_2 on the expression of genes involved in bile acid synthesis and glucose homeostasis in mice with humanized PXR. *Nutrients, 10*(8), 982. https://www.mdpi.com/2072-6643/10/8/982.

Tang, H., Zheng, Z., Wang, H., Wang, L., Zhao, G., & Wang, P. (2022, April 4). Vitamin K_2 Modulates Mitochondrial Dysfunction Induced by 6-Hydroxydopamine in SH-SY5Y Cells via Mitochondrial Quality-Control Loop. *Nutrients, 14*(7), 1504. https://doi.org/10.3390/nu14071504.

The Healthy MD. (2020, August 31). Best foods for vitamin K_2 (MK4 and MK7). *The Healthy MD.* https://thehealthymd.com/best-foods-for-vitamin-k2-mk4-and-mk7.

Tsukamoto, Y., Ichise, H., Kakuda, H., & Yamaguchi, M. et al. (2000, June). Intake of fermented soybean (natto) increases circulating vitamin K_2 (menaquinone-7) and γ-carboxylated osteocalcin concentration in normal individuals. *Journal of Bone and Mineral Metabolism; J Bone Miner Metab 18,* 216–222. https://doi.org/10.1007/s007740070023.

WebMD Editorial Contributors. (2020, October 30). Top foods high in vitamin K_2. *WebMD.* https://www.webmd.com/diet/foods-high-in-vitamin-k2.

Wen, L., Chen, J., Duan, L., & Li, S. (2018, April 27). Vitamin K-dependent proteins involved in bone and cardiovascular health (Review). *Molecular Medicine Reports; 18(1)*, 3-15. https://doi.org/10.3892/mmr.2018.8940.

Wikipedia Contributors. (2023, March 17). Vitamin K$_2$. *Wikimedia Foundation.* En.wikipedia.org. https://en.wikipedia.org/wiki/Vitamin_K2.

Chapter 7: Feasting Formula

Pitchford, P. (2009). *Healing with whole foods: Asian traditions and modern nutrition (3rd ed.).* Berkeley, Calif: North Atlantic Books.

Chapter 8: Conscious Celebration

A. (2016, September 3). Count your many blessings and it will surprise you what the Lord has done. *BibleTruths.* https://www.bibletruths.org/count-your-blessings.

Ho, L. (2023, February 3). How to celebrate small wins to achieve big goals. *Lifehack.* https://www.lifehack.org/396379/how-celebrate-small-wins-achieve-big-goals.

Hutto, C. (2020, December 8). 14 creative ways to celebrate small wins. *InHerSight.* https://www.inhersight.com/blog/career-development/celebrate-small-wins.

Kajabi. (2023, February 22). 5 ways to celebrate success and kick imposter syndrome to the curb. *RSS.* https://kajabi.com/blog/how-to-celebrate-success-at-work.

Robbins, T. (2018, January 1). 7 ways to celebrate success. *Tony Robbins.* https://www.tonyrobbins.com/mind-meaning/how-do-you-celebrate-your-success.

Rothstein, L., & Stromme, D. (n.d.). Celebrate the small stuff. *Positive Psychology | UMN Extension.* https://extension.umn.edu/two-you-video-series/celebrate-small-stuff.

The Silver Leaf Company. (2018, August 1). *Paying it forward.* https://silverleafcompany.co.za/2018/08/.

Accountability

E James Rohn. (1996). *Leading an inspired life.* Wheeling, IL: Nightingale-Conant.

ABOUT NAOMI LINDSEY

Naomi Lindsey is a busy wife, mom of five, grandmother, Wellness and Nutrition Consultant, and the author of *Intermittent Fasting for Women Over 50: The 3-Step Transformational Formula to Melt Fat in Less Than 27 Days*.

Not everyone thrives on exercise, and Naomi was one of these people. She was in love with her work as a Travel Nurse and Home Care Nurse and committed all her time to help patients and meeting deadlines. But being tied to her desk with paperwork, there was little time for her family, which caused sleepless nights—and this was when the health problems began.

The sedentary lifestyle led to weight gain that blew out of control. Naomi wasn't stupid; she knew she needed to exercise but was too scared. Even a short walk left her gasping for air. Next came various health issues that are associated with weight gain. The final straw was when her mental health started to suffer.

All of her research and professional experience pointed Naomi to intermittent fasting but never could she have imagined the full extent of the benefits this lifestyle change would bring about.

In record time, Naomi lost 123 pounds, but what amazed her more was that the weight stayed off. There was no sagging or stretched skin. Instead, her sleep improved, and she felt energized and confident, so much so that she took the calculated risk of changing her career in her 50s! As if this wasn't enough, Naomi discovered that her relationship with exercise changed, and she is now happier than ever running, playing basketball, and doing squats.

Naomi looks and feels 20 years younger, and this motivates her to help other women. The menopausal years can be horrendous. It's hard to understand the changes to a woman's body and manage the extreme symptoms. It can be a very isolating time for women, especially as menopause is still such a taboo subject.

Naomi has reached the age and stage of her life where she is in the perfect position to share the knowledge she acquired as a nurse, along with her amazing experience with intermittent fasting to improve her overall well-being.

As a consultant, Naomi has already seen how her advice and support have helped countless women. It's time to help even more women with a lifestyle change that not only works but is actually fun!

Printed in Great Britain
by Amazon